5 Stages of
Health

DR ROSS WALKER'S
5 Stages of
Health

Debunk the media myths and get the facts of good health

BANTAM

SYDNEY AUCKLAND TORONTO NEW YORK LONDON

A Bantam book
Published by Random House Australia Pty Ltd
Level 3, 100 Pacific Highway, North Sydney NSW 2060
www.randomhouse.com.au

First published by Bantam in 2012

National Library of Australia
Cataloguing-in-Publication entry: (pbk)

Walker, Ross G. T.
The five stages of health / Dr. Ross Walker.

ISBN 978 1 74275 250 1 (pbk.)

Health.
Lifestyles.

613

Cover photography by Elizabeth Allnutt
Cover design by saso content & design pty ltd
Internal design and typesetting by Midland Typesetters, Australia
Printed in Australia by Griffin Press, an accredited ISO AS/NZS 14001:2004 Environmental Management System printer

Random House Australia uses papers that are natural, renewable and recyclable products and made from wood grown in sustainable forests. The logging and manufacturing processes are expected to conform to the environmental regulations of the country of origin.

Contents

Introduction

Do you ever stop during a typical, busy day and ask yourself, 'What am I doing this for?' If you're reading this in Australia, you may recall the briefest political career in history, when the rugby league legend Mal Meninga decided to throw his hat into the political ring. During the first few questions of the press conference announcing his candidature, however, he exclaimed, 'I can't do this!'

He stood up, apologised and walked out, back to the world where he felt comfortable and in control, i.e. rugby league.

How many of you reading this feel trapped in your life? How many have constant niggles, maybe a chronic complaint, can't lose weight, feel persistently tired and often stressed?

If you ticked the box to any of these, there is something in this book for you. I am confident the vast majority of you often ask, 'What do I want out of life? How can I lead a longer, happier, more fulfilling life?'

What is wrong with our modern society that promotes this chronic state of angst and lack of wellbeing?

Over the past 20 to 30 years, we have witnessed the emergence of the 'wellness industry', offering – you guessed it – 'wellness' in its many forms.

We have seen the explosion of wellness centres, day spas, health periodicals, internet sites and a variety of products promising cures from wrinkles to Alzheimer's disease and even haemorrhoids. The medical profession is happy to support the benefits of 'lifestyle modification' but falls short of condoning the less accepted processes such as detoxification and certainly warns against the more bizarre, such as colonic washouts!

Throughout the modern world, the more affluent are spending thousands of hard-earned dollars each day on nutriceutical products, cosmetics and cosmetic procedures, hoping to look younger, feel younger, age less and live longer.

So, does any of this stuff work or is it just a sham? Should we abandon this quest for external youth and purely accept the conservative, orthodox medical view telling us all to follow a healthy lifestyle and accept your 'medical lot' when it happens; in other words, shut up and take your pills!

I must say, during my 30 years of practising medicine I've only come across a small minority of people who are truly happy, healthy and contented with their life.

Thus, the norm for our modern world is lack of wellness, fatigue, poor health and, most importantly, discontentment. One of the key elements here that I see is that we are living against our physiology.

We occasionally hear the story of a person who nurtures a lion or a tiger as a pet from birth. When the animal has matured into a fully grown beast, if something goes wrong the animal may turn against its owner and violently rip them to shreds. As tragic as this is, it certainly comes as no surprise.

Lions and tigers were not physiologically designed to be brought up living in symbiosis with human beings. Ripping another animal to shreds – humans included – is part of the job description for these big cats. Strangely, if they are hungry, cornered or angry they'll behave like a lion or tiger. Now bring in modern man. Our basic physiology hasn't really changed that much over the past 10,000 to 50,000 years. Evolution is not that rapid. We humans were designed for the following circumstances:

1. A totally natural world with exposure only to natural substances;
2. Feast and famine;
3. Constant movement;
4. The acute stress of the constant threat of attack from other humans or animals;
5. A short lifespan (average 30 years), because of the harshness of the environment.

Like it or not, this is the nature of our physiology. And with our knowledge and experience of the modern world, let's face it, living as a hunter-gatherer in a very unforgiving environment for, on average, around 30 years, would suck!

Who wants to spend their days wandering through a jungle searching for food, only to have their life cut short by an attack from a sabre-tooth tiger or some nasty infection, unresponsive to the antibiotics that weren't available anyway during that prehistoric era?

Now let's look at our modern world. We live in an environment where we are exposed to:

1. A variety of at times rather toxic, synthetic chemicals;
2. A number of different sources of electromagnetic and other forms of radiation;

3. Chronic stresses of living in the modern world;
4. A very sedentary lifestyle;
5. A longer lifespan and therefore longer exposure to all of the above.

Thus, in many ways, modern humans are living as if we were polar bears transported to the desert. So rather than being polar bears overheating under the Saharan sun, we are humans overeating under the golden arches.

But to understand why we now suffer the vast array of modern diseases, firstly we need to have a basic understanding of how the body works. There is a wonderful saying, 'As is the microcosm, so is the macrocosm.'

Each cell is a unit and the basic principles here also relate to the basic principles of how each individual organ, the entire body, a community, the earth, and even the universe function as a whole.

All the environmental exposures I've mentioned above lead to derangements in our body at a cellular level. The combination of a variety of environmental toxins in an individual's particular genetics typically leads to a specific disease.

But it's not just about diseases; it's also about living longer and living well. There is no doubt that we're all living longer. The most recent figures from the Bureau of Statistics tell us that the number of people in Australia over the age of 65 has increased from 11 per cent to 13.3 per cent in the last 20 years. In raw numbers, that's an increase of about one million people. And the number of people over the age of 85 is now over 380,000.

I'll get to the five stages of health shortly, but from a health and wellness perspective, I believe our aim should be:

1. Maintain good and consistent levels of energy;
2. Maintain physical wellbeing through keeping to ideal body weight, keeping your muscles strong and toned, and keeping up your level of fitness;
3. Ensure that you continue to think well and maintain your memory;
4. Maintain wellness through the absence of disease;
5. Live longer but also live better through all of the above.

What makes life on earth what it is, is the imperfection. The only thing certain about life is that we're all going to die at some stage. I know you're thinking, 'What about the old saying about death and taxes?' Well, even the taxes are not absolutely definite, especially if your accountant has good friends on an exotic, tax-free haven somewhere …

But we do live in an imperfect, impermanent world where things go wrong. Also, we live in an inexact world where we hear so many mixed messages and contradictions. How often do you hear one expert in any aspect of life make some discovery or emphatic comment, only to have this refuted by yet another expert? I can fully understand how the public is confused by many aspects of the medical messages that we've been bombarded with over the past 20 to 30 years.

One year, it's all about low fat, then it's no carbs and high protein. One minute, eggs are an evil, the next they're encouraged by heart foundations around the world. And every synthetic chemical under the sun has been associated with cancers, from aluminium in deodorants to peanut butter.

So, I believe it is important to examine the medical controversies. Should we be taking vitamins or do we derive all the vitamins, minerals and trace minerals we need from our food? Many members of the orthodox medical world suggest that all vitamins do is give you expensive urine. Well, I'll present evidence to you that they also give you expensive blood, which is exactly what you want.

Should you take calcium to build healthy bones or does this increase your risk of a heart attack? Is hormone replacement therapy a poison or is it of some benefit? Does the medical profession have excessive faith in the benefits of pharmaceutical drugs whilst playing down the side effects? For example, Lipitor – a cholesterol-lowering drug – is the biggest-selling drug in the world, but is it the wonder drug that many people believe? There is no doubt that pharmaceutical drugs have altered the destiny of many millions of people, but has this come at a price? I'll examine the benefits, but also the downsides, of the pharmaceutical model.

A major contentious issue in medicine is that of screening. There are a number of questions that arise from the concept of screening. Does it detect early disease in a truly accurate and predictive fashion? If you detect early disease, is there anything you can do about it? What age should screening start and what specific diseases should be screened?

Probably the most controversial and contentious issue in medicine is what will happen in the future. How often do you hear or read the news in the media about an amazing medical breakthrough, only to find out that the test, therapy or intervention is purely in the testing phase and probably won't be available for at least five to 10 years.

I have heard (and am possibly guilty of this in my own position as a media doctor) about major medical breakthroughs in every aspect of medicine, never to hear of them again, or which, when properly tested, turn out to be fizzers. The cure for cancer is always five to 10 years away and it has been five to 10 years away for the last 15 to 20 years.

I must, however, proffer my opinion that stem-cell therapy, genetic screening and genetic therapies will be the next big thing in medicine. A week rarely goes by without original articles in most major peer-review journals demonstrating their benefits.

So should we accept our lot and keep living the way we are or is there a better solution? Does the pill-procedure paradigm of the medical profession work or is there a better solution? Well, you may be surprised, but I think the answer lies somewhere in the middle. As a doctor and practising cardiologist, I am a great believer in many aspects of orthodox medicine and I believe a shunning of the medical model is foolish. If you're suffering any acute medical problem such as a heart attack, a gastrointestinal bleed or acute appendicitis (just to give a few examples), there is no better place to be than the A & E Department of any major hospital. Don't go running off to your complementary therapist for a solution to these problems because it is highly likely you won't survive. But, to take this to the next level, after your acute problem has settled, don't think you are healed. In fact, the mechanical aspects of your treatment are only just the beginning.

The five stages of health

The focus of this book is, of course, the five stages of health. In the first few chapters, I'll outline some of the hurdles standing between us and good physical and spiritual health, offering lots of tips along the way, as well as discussing the other health issues I've mentioned above. I'll go into much more detail about the actual five stages from chapter 11 onwards, but for now, here's a brief description of the stages that I believe we all need to work through in order to be truly healed:

1. **Body health**: here is where orthodox medicine is king. If you are having a heart attack, the best treatment is to have a stent (a small metal scaffold) inserted urgently across the blockage in your coronary artery. If your gall bladder is diseased and full of stones, no manner of meditation, herbs or detox will clear the problem. You need it removed!

   If your blood pressure is elevated, following all the lifestyle measures I'll mention later on will certainly help, but if it is still up, no manner of herbs, vitamins or any other complementary medications will have much effect. Blood pressure-lowering treatments are the key here.

2. **Environmental**: although we are all separate entities, we still exist in an external environment. This environment has the potential to be toxic. These toxins can exist at a microcosmic level, i.e. purely affecting the individual, or a macrocosmic level, i.e. having the potential to affect all of us.

   Two obvious examples here are smoking and pollution.

Smoking is a personal choice (and may I suggest not a particularly good one) which poisons your microcosmic environment. Pollution affects us all. If we decide to live within the confines of a larger city, pollution is an unwanted consequence of this choice. The evidence is rather telling that pollution has many dire health consequences.

Thus, it's important to clean up both your microcosmic and macrocosmic environments, as much as you can, living in this modern world.

3. **Genetic**: that wonderful old saying, 'You can pick your friends, but you can't pick your relatives,' is a very important notion in the generation of disease. Some diseases, such as Huntington's chorea, Down syndrome and a myriad of other (thankfully) uncommon conditions are purely genetic. You are born with the gene, you're stuck with the condition.

A number of other conditions, however, very much depend on the gene–environment interaction. In this situation, it is your genes that load the gun, but your environment that pulls the trigger.

It is my firm belief, backed up by numerous scientific studies, that although at this stage in the vast majority of situations we can't change your genes (but watch this space), we can alter the manifestations of the genes and thus change the natural history of your underlying condition for the better.

4. **Emotional**: unfortunately, far too often I see the person who interrupts their extremely stressful, miserable life by having an

acute medical problem, only to return to their extremely stress-ful, miserable life.

Stress, along with life crises, may be precipitating, aggravating and at times causative factors towards many of our common diseases. It is vital for health that the basic structure of your life changes under these circumstances.

5. **Mind health**: this is the most difficult and, indeed, most contentious aspect of the process of becoming healthy. This section is not provable by modern scientific techniques and is, in fact, based on thousands of years of Eastern medicine. Becoming healthy at this level is also the most confronting aspect of the five stages.

The spiritual teacher and medical intuitive Caroline Myss has written and taught on this aspect of healing and health for a number of years, which is summarised beautifully by the phrase, 'Your biography becomes your biology.'

Health is certainly not just swallowing a pill or having a medical procedure – it is a total process. I see every day as a self-improvement program: 'How can I become better in all areas of my life?'

Until you can incorporate all five stages into your life by the process detailed in this book, it is my belief you cannot be truly healthy.

PART I

CHAPTER 1

Disconnection from our true nature

As I've mentioned, historically our physiological use-by date was 30 to 40 years. Of course, the vast majority of people nowadays live beyond the age of 40 and there is no-one who looks or feels as vibrant in their later years as they did when they were younger.

It reminds me of the woman in her 60s who visits her doctor and says, 'Doctor, my face is wrinkled, my breasts are sagging, my bum's expanding and I can't get this fat off my belly.' The doctor replies, 'Well, at least the positive side here is that your vision is still working perfectly.'

So many people are rushing off to the plastic or cosmetic surgeon to have a multitude of procedures in the vain hope they can maintain a modicum of youth. Actually, it's my opinion that plastic surgery doesn't make you look better, it purely makes you look different!

Regardless of the superficial desire to maintain youthful looks and vigour, the basic human desire or instinct is survival. Our basic human fear is the fear of death, which is a logical follow on from our desire to survive.

We have evolved automatic systems within our body to aid our survival. These systems are the well-known 'fear, flight, fight' system. I prefer to call this system – which is scientifically called the sympathetic nervous system – the five F system, adding to the first three Fs, fright and that wonderful activity many of us get to enjoy, typically before going to sleep.

This system, which involves specialised nerves distributed throughout the body starting in an area of your brain called the hypothalamus, connects these nerves to your pupils to widen them to open up your field of vision, as well as your blood vessels, again to widen or dilate them to deliver more blood to your muscles and brain and also to increase your strength and alertness.

All of the above occurs when your body perceives it is in any trouble or danger or needs to rapidly put in that extra effort to perform. In prehistoric times, this allowed our ancestors to either defend themselves or run during times of attack.

We even have two paired glands sitting on either kidney which are basically our 'stress glands', known as the adrenal glands. The adrenal glands make and secrete adrenalin during times of acute stress, as well as cortisone (and related compounds) during more chronic stresses.

That's why, when you suddenly become frightened, you experience those butterflies in your stomach. It is actually the release of adrenalin from your adrenal glands and not you inadvertently swallowing an insect.

The opposing system is known as the parasympathetic system or the five Rs – rest, rejuvenation, relaxation, revival, restart. I know I am stretching it here – especially if you own a thesaurus (incidentally, did you know there is no other word for thesaurus!) – but I am obligated to maintain the 'five' theme. If I monitored your pulse, blood pressure and blood flow to your organs during very deep sleep, your entire system would be slowed right down. Your five Rs would have kicked right in to prepare your body for the onslaught of the next day. The last thing you need in the middle of a deep sleep is your heart jumping out of your chest and torrential blood flow to your muscles and organs.

You can see that both systems are very much geared to survival – the sympathetic nervous system to protect you in times of danger and the parasympathetic nervous system to conserve energy and repair you to ensure you survive longer and better.

Both systems also demonstrate the true secret to a quality long life, i.e. balance. This is the middle path between the extremes of danger and relaxation. In physiologic terms, we call this homeostasis. As your cells, organs, brain and the rest of your physical body constantly strive for this balance, so should you in all aspects of your life. (Again repeating a theme: as is the microcosm, so is the macrocosm.)

The most successful people in our modern world try to achieve this balance:

1. Physically
2. Emotionally
3. Mentally
4. Work life
5. Spiritually

In this book, I will explain the keys to achieving balance in all of these categories.

Another important system that is geared towards our survival is the pleasure centre. There are five basic human needs that promote survival:

1. The need for nutrition through food and fluid
2. The need for adequate shelter to protect us against the elements
3. The need for social interaction
4. The need to procreate to ensure parts of our DNA survive once we have shuffled off this mortal coil
5. The need to acquire knowledge, from the more basic survival skills to obtain some of the above, to the more intricate emotional and cognitive skills which strengthen the quality of all of the above.

There is a set of 'feel-good' chemicals that is released into various parts of the brain when any of these needs are met. There is a centre deep within our brain, the nucleus accumbens (our pleasure centre). When this is stimulated, a chemical – dopamine – is released that gives us that wonderful feeling of pleasure.

This centre evolved in the time we were hunter-gatherers so that we had appropriate dopamine release when we ate nurturing food, felt warm and safe and protected from the elements, or interacted with our families. And (as I'm sure you'd imagine) there is a fair whack of dopamine released into the nucleus accumbens each time we have an orgasm.

Also, we've all experienced that 'ah-hah' moment when we learn a new skill or have an extraordinary idea, with the accompanying burst of dopamine to enhance the experience.

Closely linked to the nucleus accumbens–dopamine network is the endorphin system, which is your body's natural opiates. Basically, stimulation of the nucleus accumbens occurs more during a rush of excitement, whereas when endorphins are released they tend to induce that feeling of dreamy satisfaction. Although not as straightforward as this, it basically works this way.

A major problem in our modern world is that we have discovered creative and very destructive ways to stimulate our pleasure system. For instance, stimulants such as cocaine and ecstasy hijack the nucleus accumbens, and excessive use can permanently damage the area to the point where the only method of stimulating this centre is with the use of these illegal substances. It only takes one hit of crack (freebase cocaine) to induce this damage and thus instant addiction.

All forms of addiction are linked to damage in one of these systems, creating the ongoing need for whatever is the source of your addiction.

But it doesn't have to be an illegal drug that hijacks these systems. Any excess, which may involve overeating, gambling, alcohol or any type of aberrant behaviour, can lead to this issue. Of course, it would be remiss of me not to give a special mention to that legal and very serious addiction, cigarette smoking.

This all reinforces my concept that we are disconnected from our true nature in this society.

So, let's go back in time before time was actually invented. Over 10,000 years ago we were purely hunter-gatherers, at the top of the food chain, where you knew you'd had a good day if all your limbs were intact and you weren't bleeding from somewhere after a bad interaction with a potential competing food source.

Let's examine a day in the life of a hunter-gatherer. Let's call him Grunt. Grunt and his devoted wife, Gruntina, live with their two children, a boy, Grunter, and his baby sister, Gruntel. (Yes, the names were unimaginative back in those days as language hadn't been discovered.)

Grunt drags himself off the cave floor as the first light streams through the entrance. Gruntina stirs as her husband forages around in the semi-darkness for his electric razor. As you can imagine, the absence of the shaving apparatus from the prehistoric environment meant Grunt wasted a lot of time looking for his shaver. After accepting the presence of his extremely long beard, pulling on his rudimentary clothes he ventures off to find some food for his family to fill their rather empty bellies.

Hopefully, he arrives back with some food which needs to be consumed immediately because the pantry and the fridge typically don't work that well.

Once the sun sets there is not much to do apart from that horizontal activity many of us enjoy – yes, sleeping is what I'm referring to! As there are many more hours of night than day, sleeping occupies much of their time. Also the television was even worse than it is today!

This was their daily existence until that inevitable attack from a bigger, quicker predator, or a just as devastating assault from an unseen microbe, which muscled in on one of their organs, bludgeoning their immune system into submission.

Thus, the major killers of the hunter-gatherer world were trauma and infection. These days, when we typically live much longer, our parts start to wear out. And for all us men over 50, everything stiffens up apart from the bits you want to.

Here, then, are the three rules of being a male over 50:

1. Never walk past a public convenience
2. Never waste an erection
3. Never trust a fart!

From a health viewpoint, the major issue we're confronted with is that although our world has changed dramatically since the days we were hunter-gatherers, our physiology hasn't really changed that much. Let's examine each feature of how this physiology is supposed to behave:

1. Fuelled by natural substances: in the hunter-gatherer world, fuel and food were consumed purely for survival; these days, we see consumption of these substances as one of life's pleasures. Of course, as I have already argued, the hunter-gatherers derived pleasure from the consumption of food; if not, they wouldn't have spent the majority of their days wandering around inhospitable environments to obtain the stuff.

    To reinforce my point, all of our positive behaviours and physiologies are geared towards this survival. But we humans are lazy devils, and with our need to acquire knowledge this acquisition has led us to develop shortcuts to obtain this stimulation and pleasure. These shortcuts can be anything from excessive use of food, alcohol or illegal substances, to jumping out of planes, preferably with a parachute firmly attached to our backs.

2. Feast and famine: the hunter-gatherer physiology was certainly adapted to the feast of the kill. If you didn't consume your kill immediately or eat the vegetables once they were plucked from their source, it didn't take long for the food supply to go off. But there were numerous times when the hunter would arrive back at the cave empty-handed. (The other animals also had strong survival mechanisms, so they didn't volunteer their services freely as a steady source of nourishment.)

Thus, ancient man evolved a number of mechanisms to maintain survival during these times of famine. Also, coinciding with this lack of food was a lack of fluid. Of course, lack of food and fluid leads to lack of water and salt and thus dehydration. Dehydration leads to reduced blood flow to the vital organs; in particular, the brain, the heart and the kidneys. Unless this is corrected, the organs lose their function and eventually fail.

A vital mechanism developed to cope with these times of dehydration is known as the renin-angiotensin system. When this system is switched on, it releases chemicals that constrict blood vessels that prop up the blood pressure and retains salt and water.

Another important mechanism here is the ability to store fat during times of reduced food supply. These fat stores held a small supply of fat around the hunter-gatherer belly to provide energy during times of starvation. We have three sources of macronutrients – fat, sugar and protein – all of which are needed for appropriate delivery of energy for the body: an absolute necessity for survival.

Once the body goes into starvation mode, it switches into a state of catabolism – in other words, the breakdown of normal structures – which leads to breakdown of fat stores, protein from muscle and the release of sugars from what is known as the glycogen stores in the liver and muscle. The fat stores are the most efficient energy stores.

There is a common condition called insulin resistance (which I'll explain in greater depth later) that decreases the free entry of nutrients, especially into the muscles. If you have insulin resistance, the fat is stored around the belly to be used during these times of famine, and also sugar levels are somewhat higher, which keeps the brain more active during these times.

The brain really only functions correctly with adequate sugar; the other fuels (such as fat) don't really work. Thus, insulin resistance was an extraordinary advantage as a hunter-gatherer, but is a major disadvantage in our modern world, as you'll see later.

At a micronutrient level, i.e. vitamins, minerals and trace metals, the body also developed mechanisms to maintain survival. One of the major mechanisms here was a cholesterol-carrying protein known as Lipoprotein(a). Lp(a) initially evolved during prolonged starvation states to counteract the reduced intake of vitamin C. Human beings are one of only four animal species which cannot metabolise their own vitamin C and thus we must obtain it from food sources, typically citrus fruits.

The water-soluble vitamins (such as B group and vitamin C) need to be taken daily because they are not stored well in the body. The fat-soluble vitamins (A, D, E and K) are stored (strangely) in fat and thus hang around for longer. Think of it logically – water is fluid and flows away quickly; fat is solid and gluggy, slow moving, and holds on to stuff.

Vitamin C is a vital component of collagen, which keeps our blood vessels and other supporting structures flexible and functioning normally. If there isn't a constant supply of this vitamin in your system, your supporting structures (including the blood vessels) become weak.

A simple message: eat fruit, especially citrus, in some form every day and it doesn't hurt to top this up with a vitamin C supplement.

In the days of the hunter-gatherer, the two to three day trek from one eating hole to the next often meant a few days without reasonable nutrition, leading to an acute drop in water-soluble vitamins, including vitamin C.

Vitamin C deficiency, otherwise known as scurvy, is characterised by weak blood vessels that break down and thus bleed. Bleeding into the gums and subcutaneous tissues is a common manifestation of this condition.

Professor Linus Pauling, who won two unshared Nobel Prizes, proposed – along with his colleague Matthias

Rath – that lipoprotein Lp(a) was involved as an antidote to the intermittent periods of vitamin C deficiency experienced by hunter-gatherers. Lp(a) is an LDL molecule (bad cholesterol) hooked up to an apoprotein – a chemical that actually thickens the blood. Their hypothesis was that Lp(a) plugged the holes in the blood vessels caused by the vitamin C deficiency.

Another important survival mechanism was eating fresh vegetables with adequate B group vitamins. Each component of the B vitamin family has various vital functions within the cell. In particular, adequate combinations of B6, B12 and folic acid are vital for cell repair.

The hunter-gatherer diet, which was rich in both B and C vitamins from the ingestion of fresh off-the-tree or vine fruits and vegetables, ensured very high doses of B group vitamins for adequate cell repair. However, this only occurred during the times of plenty, and unfortunately, especially during a harsh winter, these fruits and vegetables were often not available. This created weakness in the hunter-gatherer's immune system and susceptibility to infection.

3. Constant movement: sitting in your cave all day wasn't really an adequate method of finding or hunting for food. So, a major feature of the hunter-gatherer existence was constant movement to hunt and gather food. (Thus, the name.)

Without constant movement, which included evading other rather large and ferocious animals that saw *you* as their food source, the hunter-gatherer would soon perish. So, our bodies were designed to be moving machines. You were designed to have fluid, toned muscles that could snap into action at the drop of a ferocious-looking jaw from an unexpected place.

4. Acute stress: the only stress our body was designed for was the acute stress of the kill or acute danger to ourselves, as well as another rather obvious stress and danger – the need to stave off infections.

Generally, the two major causes of death in the world of the hunter-gatherer were trauma and infection. Thus, two systems evolved which were basically geared to protect us against these two probable events.

i. Clotting–bleeding axis: I've already mentioned the vital concept of balance. All the feedback systems in our body are geared to keep us somewhere in the middle to maintain our normal physiology.

None can be more vital than the clotting–bleeding axis. If our blood was too thick, it would be difficult for the heart and circulation to maintain smooth flow through the arteries and veins. Sluggish, thick blood would clot very easily, leading to premature death from heart attack, stroke and venous thrombosis.

But, if our blood was too 'thin', we'd bleed to death from any minor trauma or abrasion. Women wouldn't survive through any menstrual period. So, our body getting that balance right is crucial.

ii. The immune system: the only reason microbes haven't totally dominated the world is because of the development of a powerful immune system in the animal kingdom. This immune system is very much geared to fight all foreign proteins. There are very effective antibodies and immune cells in our body that mount a defence response against bacteria, fungi and viruses.

At an emotional level, the hunter-gatherer's feelings were very simplistic and reactive. Their emotions allowed them to love and nurture their offspring and to generate anger when they or their loved ones were in danger. They lived in the moment, without much in the way of future planning.

Now let's bring in the modern world:

1. Synthetic chemicals: although nature hasn't been completely destroyed, many of the natural chemicals and foods used by hunter-gatherers have been altered in ways to make them last longer, look better, taste better (some would say), and will be used for anything from washing and making you smell better to ridding the body or surfaces of unwanted bugs.

    The problem here is that we were not designed to be exposed to the variety of synthetic chemicals so widespread in our modern world. These chemicals are a major factor in many of our modern diseases.

2. Radiation: various types of subtle and not so subtle forms of radiation are a common feature of our modern existence. It's estimated that the average person living in any modern

community is exposed to around the radiation equivalent of five chest x-rays per year.

This is purely from all manner of electronic appliances, including computers and mobile phones. It's well established that excessive radiation exposure is not particularly good for the body.

3. Sedentary lifestyle with a constant food supply: this is a recipe for obesity. In the modern world you're not saving up those fat stores for a 'starvy' day; you're basically piling up the layers with continual eating and not much movement.

4. Chronic stresses: from the moment you're woken up in the morning (strangely, it's called an *alarm* clock – even the language is stressful) to the moment you wake up the next morning, modern living can be one dose of stress after the other. Rushing to get ready for work; the long commute; deadlines; office politics; annoying, demanding bosses; lazy, incompetent workers – and I haven't even started on the complexities of modern families.

Unfortunately, many of these chronic stresses contribute to the state of constant unhappiness many people experience in the modern environment.

5. Longer life/longer exposure: because we're living longer than the hunter-gatherer, we're exposed to all of the unnatural factors for a much longer period.

Probably the biggest factor we avoid by all of these distractions in the modern world is: why? Why are we here? What is our true purpose? I believe we are unhappy because we feel so disconnected from our true nature, our true self, our true sense of purpose. There is this wonderful saying about 'climbing the ladder to success to find you're on the wrong wall'. How many of us are on the wrong wall and what can we do about it? Read on.

CHAPTER 2

Our modern killers

Cardiovascular disease

The famous actor and film director Woody Allen once commented, 'It's not that I'm afraid of death – I just don't want to be there when it happens.' For the vast majority, though – all of us, really – when your number is up, it's up.

Since we've arrived on this planet well over 10,000 years too late, it's highly likely we won't die from that sabre-toothed tiger attack, although we may succumb to some nasty infection. The number one cause of death in modern society is cardiovascular disease in all its forms. Biting at its heels – and certainly not too far behind – is the ever-increasing problem of cancer.

Cardiovascular disease accounts for around 45 per cent of deaths in the modern world. The central and most important factor is atherosclerosis. Atherosclerosis is the progressive build-up of fat and other gunk in the wall of your arteries, which occurs from a very early age. This has been found in the arteries of some newborn babies whose mothers smoked or had big-league cholesterol problems, and it typically starts when you begin ingesting baby food, which is full of synthetic fats and other muck.

Hunter-gatherers, who spent their time finding food and avoiding being the main course for the larger members of the animal kingdom, did not have enough fat in their system for the excess to spill into the walls.

But in our modern world of abundant food and a sedentary lifestyle, as well as excess salt, our cholesterol levels easily rise above three milli-mole per litre and our blood pressure is typically above 100 millimetres of mercury, so any excess fat or pressure promotes fat build-up in the walls. If you imagine a donut (which will also become relevant later), there is a large hole in the middle, but all the action is happening in the wall. It's the same for atherosclerosis. Fat builds up in the wall without causing blockage, but if this suddenly ruptures, a clot forms over the rupture leading to a heart attack, stroke or sudden death, depending on the size and location of the rupture.

This is precisely why an executive stress test is not a reliable predictor for future vascular risk. Your artery may be nice and open whilst you are performing the test, despite a huge fatty plaque sitting in the wall of the artery just waiting for the opportunity to suddenly burst and form that potentially fatal clot.

This process is not just a cholesterol phenomenon, but actually depends on a combination of several components.

Endothelial dysfunction

If I asked you the Trivial Pursuit question, 'What is the biggest organ in the body?', those of you who were not in the know would probably say the heart, the liver or possibly the brain, and you would be wrong.

The Trivial Pursuit answer is the skin. The skin is an actively functioning organ and is larger in area and volume than all the other major organs in the body. However, this is, in fact, the wrong answer. The biggest organ in the body is the endothelium, which is a single layer of cells that covers every blood vessel in the body. This is also an actively functioning organ in that, not only does it act as a barrier to stop the blood running through it leaking across into the blood vessel wall, it also secretes very important substances that maintain balanced blood flow to different organs.

There is a ubiquitous vasodilator (blood vessel opener) known as nitric oxide. There is also the counter-balancing chemical known as endothelin, which constricts blood vessels. In a healthy person, these two chemicals are very important. When you are exercising, moving or are experiencing fear, it is very important you have an excellent blood flow to your heart and all of your other organs, and thus signals are sent to a healthy endothelium to release nitric oxide. On the other hand, when you are in a deep sleep in the middle of the night rejuvenating your body, the last thing you need is torrential blood flow to your muscles and the major organs and thus endothelin is secreted to conserve energy and not waste your precious resources so you can be rejuvenated for the next day.

If you ask most people what causes heart attacks, you'll get answers like high cholesterol, high blood pressure, cigarette smoking etc. But the first step in the generation of heart disease is malfunction of the endothelium. This is not caused by having a high cholesterol level, but is due to synthetic chemicals, radiation and chronic stresses damaging the endothelium and allowing the altered LDL cholesterol – bad cholesterol – to cross the damaged endothelium and set up shop in the wall of your arteries.

To just look at total cholesterol levels or blood pressure by itself is far too simplistic; so, in the first instance, it is important to maintain a healthy endothelium. Mind you, all of the traditional risk factors for heart disease may contribute to damaging the endothelium. For example, it has been shown clearly that a great cause of injury to the endothelium is smoking cigarettes. There are now ways to assess endothelial function and numerous studies have demonstrated that the endothelium is already performing poorly in teenage and young adult smokers.

FIVE STEPS TO STRENGTHEN YOUR ENDOTHELIUM

1. Minimise exposure to synthetic chemicals, radiation and chronic stresses.

2. Maintain a healthy natural diet with good doses of plant chemicals.

3. L-Arginine – the precursor step to the generation of nitric oxide is L-Arginine. This is a specific amino acid that must be obtained from the diet, as your body cannot make it internally. Five major scientific studies have shown that eating 10 to 15 nuts per day reduces cardiovascular risk by around 50 per cent. Apart from the excellent high-quality fats in nuts, there is also an abundance of L-Arginine. All high-quality proteins have some L-Arginine, but it is particularly concentrated in nuts. For those of you in significant need of a very healthy endothelium, you can also purchase L-Arginine from a health food store and take this, usually in doses of around 2–3 grams per day.

4. Cocoa – the chemical in cocoa is known as *Theobroma cacao*, which is also found in dark chocolate. Dark chocolate is abundant in what is known as flavonoid antioxidants and they have a specific effect in generating nitric oxide and have another vasodilating (blood vessel opening) substance known as prostacyclin. Trials showed that after six weeks of ingesting dark chocolate or a sugar-free cocoa, there was around a 75 per cent increase in the function of the endothelium, but this was not so dramatic when the sugar was part of the cocoa.

5. Pomegranate – the active ingredient in a pomegranate is known as *Punica granatum*, which again has profound effects on elevating nitric oxide levels. It has also been shown that people who have 125 millilitres of pomegranate juice per day have a marked increase in antioxidant status, reducing LDL oxidation (I'll explain more about antioxidants later), and around a 20 per cent drop in blood pressure.

FATS
It's not all about cholesterol

Armed with your total fat profile results, it is important that you have a basic understanding of how these should be interpreted. Firstly, I would like to make a major point which is not particularly well known or discussed by the medical profession. It is not just your cholesterol level that counts but the quality of each component.

To simplify things, this is how fats work in the body. There are bad cholesterols – which, as I've mentioned, are also known as LDLs – and good cholesterols, better known as HDLs.

However this is too simplistic, because two individuals can have quite similar LDL and HDL levels, not to mention other similar risk factors for cardiovascular disease (cigarettes, blood pressure, diabetes, etc), but one might have rampant vascular disease, whilst the other has nothing much at all. Here is where the problem lies!

What is the answer? I believe that just examining the absolute levels of cholesterol, LDL or HDL and basic treatment strategies commonly accepted by orthodox medicine leads to a number of people being over-treated with unnecessary medications, with all of their potential risks, while a number of people are not being treated and miss out on appropriate therapy. It is not just the level but the function of that particular molecule that is important.

To give an analogy – take two groups of ten men of the same age, height and body weight and ask them to complete a particular task, such as digging a trench. One group of these supposedly equally matched men might be diligent, hard working and dedicated to finishing the task efficiently within a particular timeframe. Meanwhile, the other group might be a bunch of lazy loafers who couldn't be bothered, and the job does not get finished.

Increasing research is showing that in the same fashion, not all cholesterol molecules between different individuals are created equal and have different functionality. So, just lowering LDL cholesterol by whatever means available (e.g. statin drugs) or raising HDL cholesterol (e.g. red wine, exercise, weight loss, giving up smoking or nicotinic acid) may not work for everyone.

Treatment of cholesterol abnormalities, whether with lifestyle modification or not, really depends on your level of cardiovascular risk.

TREAT CARDIOVASCULAR RISK, NOT CHOLESTEROL LEVELS

If your estimated cardiovascular risk is below 10 per cent over 10 years, drugs are not required, regardless of your cholesterol levels.

If your risk is 10 to 20 per cent, drug treatment should be given based on individual profiles, e.g. family history, presence of diabetes etc.

If your risk is greater than 20 per cent, then you require aggressive cholesterol lowering which, in most cases, will also mean some form of medications, typically statin drugs.

The greatest risk for heart disease is having already suffered heart disease in the first place. What I mean by this is that if you take two individuals, the same age, with the same cholesterol levels, the same blood pressure and family history, but one has already had a heart problem and the other has not, then the one with the previous heart problem is around 10 times more likely to suffer a further problem.

Following on from this is the more formalised issue of cardiovascular risk assessments. Over 50 years ago, a very insightful researcher in the United States, Thomas Royle Dawber, decided to observe and record the health and living habits of a relatively small community near Boston, known as Framingham.

The Framingham Heart Study examined multiple aspects of this community and the impact of a variety of parameters – cholesterol, blood pressure etc – on people's subsequent health issues. Much of our early understanding of cholesterol and blood pressure arose from this study. There is now a very well accepted term known as the Framingham Risk Score, which takes into account your cholesterol levels (both good and bad), blood pressure, whether you're a smoker or non-smoker, the presence or absence of diabetes and, of course, those two uncontrollable risk factors of age and sex.

From this information the calculated 10-year risk can be assessed. There are now numerous spin-offs of the Framingham Risk Score which can calculate your cardiac risk. My best advice here is to Google 'cardiac risk score', find a questionnaire from one of the many available websites (e.g. American Heart Association, New Zealand Risk Score Calculator etc) and calculate your own risk.

Regardless of the specific tool you use, it is generally accepted that this assessment can reasonably place you into one of the following three categories:

low risk: less than 10 per cent 10-year risk,
intermediate risk: 10 to 20 per cent 10-year risk,
high risk: greater than 20 per cent 10-year risk.

This is an important distinction, because what group you are in will then determine the aggressiveness of your need for medical investigation and treatment.

As a general rule, low-risk people only need minimal cardiac investigations and treatment. If you're in the intermediate-risk group, it is really a decision for you and your doctor as to how far you should be investigated and treated. If you're in the high-risk category, I strongly advise that you receive very aggressive medical management.

A number of experts in the field think more in terms of lifelong risk rather than 10-year risk. If you examine any individual's lifelong risk of a cardiac event, the average risk is around 45 per cent, and in higher-risk categories into the 60 to 70 per cent range. This, however, doesn't take into consideration what stage of life the person is at. In fact, as you age, your risk increases dramatically.

So, if you use the argument of lifelong risk, you'd start children on statin drugs to lower their cholesterol and also begin blood pressure treatment, which is obviously absurd. This is why I believe that we should be evaluated at a reasonably intensive level every 10 years, based on our initial risk calculations. Obviously those at intermediate and higher risk should be evaluated more often. I'd like to repeat that I don't treat cholesterol levels specifically, but treat absolute 10-year cardiac risk based on an overall assessment of the human being sitting in front of me.

CASE HISTORY

A couple of months ago, I was contacted by a senior political figure in his early 50s, reporting that he'd had some chest pain when walking up a slight hill the day before. I was concerned enough by the nature of his symptoms to suggest that he urgently obtain a referral and come to my practice immediately. The politician's story was convincing enough for me to perform an urgent stress echocardiogram (which is an ultrasound of the heart, before and after a treadmill exercise test). His exercise capacity was very poor and he developed some chest pain after only a few minutes of exercise.

His echocardiogram immediately after the test showed a moderate-sized area of lack of movement in the inferior wall of his heart, suggesting he had a blockage in his right coronary artery.

I admitted him to hospital straight away where one of my colleagues performed an angiogram, and by the afternoon the politician was back on the ward with a stent having opened his blocked right coronary artery.

I tell this story to make a few important points. Firstly, there is not a month that goes by when we don't hear of the sudden death or rapid demise of some high-profile person. Recently, in Australia, we heard of the premature death of the mobile-phone retailer John Ilhan (of 'Crazy John' fame), who died suddenly at the age of 42. It's my feeling that almost no-one dies without some sort of warning.

In a study of 22 squash players who'd died suddenly playing squash, 21 out of 22 had complained to either a doctor or relative in the week before of some type of chest pain.

The politician's case presents some very interesting facts. This man is a personal friend of mine and knows me well enough to ring me directly to discuss his problems. But how many people out there aren't personal friends with a cardiologist and develop symptoms, only to diagnose them as indigestion or ignore them because they settled as soon as they stopped exercising?

This man received what I'd like to suggest is ideal medicine. He was very lucky, but how many people don't receive ideal medicine? I know, for example, that my waiting list is now around two months, and often less proactive people go to their GP, obtain a referral, and they're booked to see any of the busy cardiologists throughout the world a few months after the initial symptoms. In many cases this is far too late.

If you've experienced chest discomfort and are not sure of the cause, this requires urgent evaluation.

There's an old saying that we're all familiar with, that the squeaky wheel gets the oil. If you suffer significant symptoms, make sure you are the 'squeaky wheel'.

BLOOD PRESSURE
Keep the pressure down!

Our old friends the hunter-gatherers evolved with arteries that were supposed to tolerate maximum blood pressures of around 95 to 100mmHg. If you examine the blood pressures of the five or so remaining hunter-gatherer races on the planet, these are precisely their readings.

In modern society things are quite different, basically because we are born into a 'sea of salt' called our mother's uterus. Salt draws fluid into the blood vessel walls, increasing the tone and therefore the pressure. In a hunter-gatherer society, the peak daily intake of salt is around the 2 gram level, but in our society, even if we restrict salt by avoiding it on our foods, in cooking, and salty foods in general, we're still probably taking in somewhere between 4 to 6 grams of salt per day. And in New Orleans, for instance, a city where hypertension – high blood pressure – is rampant, the average inhabitant consumes around 25 grams of salt per day.

Over the age of 50, hypertension is a much more important risk factor for AVD (atherosclerotic vascular disease) than cholesterol.

In the hunter-gatherer days, we evolved a set of genes that would prop our blood pressure up during times of famine and dehydration. These genes kept the blood pressure high enough so that we didn't collapse during long treks from watering hole to watering hole, with little salt or water.

Now enter our modern world where we don't suffer famine or dehydration. When we're hungry we eat and when we're thirsty we drink. Because of the excessive salt in our diet we start our lives with systolic blood pressures (top reading) that are in the 95 to 100 range and as we age (especially greater than age 50) our blood pressure usually steadily rises.

Ninety per cent of the high blood pressure seen in modern society is due to a combination of your genes in this environment. If you were taken out of the modern world at birth and put into a traditional society where there was no salt, stress or synthetic chemicals, despite having the gene for high blood pressure you would almost certainly not develop hypertension.

Ten per cent of people with hypertension have a secondary cause such as a disorder of the kidneys, adrenal glands – the two stress glands that sit on your kidneys – or a variety of rare conditions that sometimes affect the blood vessels.

If your high blood pressure is outside the normal demographic of a middle-aged or elderly person with a family history and your blood pressure is becoming increasingly difficult to control despite normal medications, then you should have a thorough screen for secondary hypertension.

Even then, the commonest cause of difficult-to-control hypertension is not some weird secondary cause, but is usually related to some form of significant life stress or excesses in other areas, such as dietary excesses with salt and alcohol or, especially in younger people, illegal drugs, such as cocaine and ecstasy.

A full and proper history from a competent doctor can usually determine whether your hypertension is due to the typical common genetic factors (often compounded by excessive life stresses) or whether you may be a potential candidate for a secondary cause.

Once you have commenced antihypertensive treatment, this is typically for life. So you should try to adopt the following five principles before you have to start medications:

1. Lose weight – even modest weight loss of between 5 to 10 kilograms can have a profound effect on reducing blood pressure.
2. Physical exercise – even without any weight loss whatsoever, regular physical exercise (at least two to three hours per week) can have almost the same effect as a blood pressure pill in dropping your blood pressure.
3. Salt restriction – even if restricting your salt doesn't drop your blood pressure, it will certainly assist in your blood pressure not continuing to rise throughout your life. It will make whatever medications you're using more effective and you should consider it a vital part of managing most cases of hypertension.
4. Alcohol restriction – although I've long been an advocate of people who enjoy drinking, having two small glasses of red wine on a daily basis, there is no doubt that once you regularly go over this level your blood pressure will elevate in a significant majority of cases. If you're serious about being healthy, any excess alcohol should never be condoned. The total daily dose suggested is 250 millilitres of wine – preferably red wine.
5. Stress management – techniques for managing stress are discussed later in the book.

There are some important points to be made about drug therapy in general and, in particular, the treatment of blood pressure. I'm always amused when a person comes to see me, delighted that their cholesterol levels have dropped to 3.5 on pharmaceutical treatment, while their blood pressure is still sitting at 160/100. If you have hypertension, it's vital that you aim for levels consistently below 135/85, and ideally in the 110 to 120 on 70 to 80 range. In almost all cases, this can be achieved with a combination of appropriate non-pharmacologic methods, such as the five mentioned above, along with targeted blood pressure treatment.

If I line up 100 people and treat them with the same blood pressure drug, only 50 will achieve adequate control on one drug. It is my experience that around half the people with high blood pressure will need anywhere between two to five drugs. Although this seems excessive, the worst approach is to allow people to have persistent elevations in their blood pressure. Over years of having poorly controlled blood pressure, the arteries thicken up and become stiff, thus contributing to all manner of cardiovascular disease.

Treating cholesterol is very uni-dimensional. People with high cholesterol levels may develop fat build-up in the walls of their arteries, but not on all occasions. The point is that cholesterol is overemphasised and over-treated, whereas blood pressure is much more important and often under-treated.

Poorly controlled hypertension, however, is very multi-dimensional and can lead to anything from cerebral haemorrhage, stroke, heart failure, atrial fibrillation and kidney disease to the biggest killer in our modern world, atherosclerosis.

Again, if I line up 100 people with high blood pressure and give them one drug, 90 will respond well to the drug whereas 10 will suffer side effects. The general side effect rate for most drugs is about 10 per cent and these can be anything from annoying, irritating side effects to very rare, severe reactions. This is why it's very important that once you commence any treatments you have regular follow-up with your doctor. It's also very important that you report immediately any new symptoms or problems that may arise after you begin treatment.

There are a number of different medication groups and it is likely that, if you have a problem with one drug from one group, you'll have a similar problem with another drug from the same group. To give you some common examples of the different types of blood pressure medications and the common side effects:

1. ACE inhibitors – 10 per cent of people experience a dry, irritating cough.
2. A2 inhibitors – minimal side effects but again occasionally a cough; also occasionally the typical drug side effects such as nausea, diarrhoea, constipation or skin rash.
3. Beta blockers – the big one here is asthma and shortness of breath. It is my practice not to use beta blockers for someone with a history of significant asthma, as beta blockers certainly have the potential to make asthma so much worse. Tiredness, depression and, in males, erectile dysfunction are potential symptoms of beta blockade. Another unusual symptom is bizarre dreams.
4. Diuretics – in the old days with very high-dose diuretic therapy, significant metabolic abnormalities such as a rise in blood sugar

level, an increased uric acid, erectile dysfunction for males and the inevitable significant loss of potassium were commonly seen. These days, diuretics are used in much lower doses and thankfully have fewer side effects.

5. Calcium channel blockers – there are various types of calcium channel blockers. Depending on the type, common symptoms are constipation, leg swelling, headache and dizziness.

There are numerous other different types of blood pressure treatments and certainly a few new drugs in the pipeline. Regardless, by working closely with your trusted medical adviser, it is almost always possible to achieve excellent blood pressure control and I must stress how vital this is for the long-term management of your atherosclerotic heart disease.

Clotting – the clot thickens

Somebody sitting in a plane from Sydney to London in the economy section, who arrives at Heathrow Airport with a deep venous thrombosis, might attempt to sue the airline. But, in reality, they should be suing their parents.

If you have a personal history of thrombosis, especially if this has occurred before the age of 55, even with circumstances of immobilisation – such as prolonged trips around the time of an operation or an injury – it is highly likely that you suffer one of the common genetic thrombotic conditions.

The majority of people have a balanced clotting-versus-bleeding system. A small but definite proportion of the population are clotters, while a lesser number of the population are, in fact, bleeders.

In almost all cases a tendency to clotting is due to a number of relatively common clotting disorders. A blood test screening for these conditions can be performed which then allows your doctor to direct appropriate blood-thinning treatment.

After the clot has been initially dissolved with intravenous or subcutaneous blood-thinning treatment, a period of time on warfarin is usually necessary. In most cases, it is then possible to switch over to oral aspirin as a preventative agent.

It is my feeling that almost all patients with coronary artery disease should be on some form of blood-thinning therapy (at least aspirin) and this decision should be an individual decision based on the nature of your heart disease.

Should all people over a certain age take aspirin?

There has been a strong school of thought to suggest that all males over 45 to 50 and all females 55 to 60 should be taking aspirin to help prevent heart disease and strokes. However, while some of the studies have been positive in this regard, none have ever shown a distinct mortality benefit, i.e. that taking aspirin or a similar drug will make you live longer. The reason for this is that around 20 per cent of the population have a tendency to bleeding. I am not suggesting that 20 per cent of the population are haemophiliacs or suffer some other serious genetic bleeding disorder, but there are certainly people who bruise easily and bleed more readily after injury or some medical or dental procedure.

I often tell the story of my mother, who took it upon herself to begin taking aspirin regularly in her early 70s. Not long afterwards, she arrived at my house for a holiday and was quite short of breath.

When I ran some tests on her, I found that she had lost half her blood volume, despite no real symptoms apart from the shortness of breath and fatigue.

On further evaluation, she'd developed a severe gastritis, almost certainly due to the aspirin therapy. After she stopped taking aspirin and was given iron, after a few months her blood returned to normal.

Therefore, taking aspirin as a preventative if you don't have a history of heart disease or haven't been deemed to be at high risk for heart disease has to be a careful decision between yourself and your doctor – not something you do yourself purely because you've heard it's a good idea. But recent studies have shown that taking a daily aspirin may reduce your heart attack and stroke rate by around 25 per cent, along with a 30 per cent reduction in many of the common cancers, so if you are not a bleeder or don't have a history of reflux, dyspepsia or ulcer problems, once you've reached 50 years of age it's a good idea to take 100mg of aspirin per day.

Inflammation – the fire within

It's not just cholesterol, doc! The new kid on the block, so to speak, is inflammation. We have a system in our body known as the immune system. This is the security guard of the body that travels around looking for damage, foreign invaders and basically trying to stop trouble before it happens. The immune system can be switched on by a number of mechanisms, one of them being a low-to-medium grade chronic infection. In recent years, a test known as 'highly sensitive C-reactive protein' (hsCRP) has been developed, which is a non-specific, but very sensitive test for the degree of inflammation in your body. If your immune system is working efficiently, you'll have a CRP less than 1.5 milligrams per decilitre. A number of studies have suggested that if your CRP is above two, and especially above three, your risk increases for some form of vascular disease.

There is no doubt that the statin drugs also have anti-inflammatory properties and moderate dose statins can reduce inflammation in the 30 to 40 per cent range. It's my opinion that an hsCRP should be part of every routine assessment. I also believe that if your hsCRP is above 1.5mg per cent, you should also be taking an anti-inflammatory dose of fish oil – at least 4000mg per day.

There are some other natural anti-inflammatories that are derived from the cruciferous vegetables, such as broccoli, cabbage and cauliflower, and I believe that we should see inflammation as an important part of the generation of AVD. Its suppression is also proving important in the management of AVD.

CASE STUDY – SUDDEN DEATH

Recently, on a cold Saturday afternoon, I turned up to play my weekly game of competition soccer. Expecting the usual enjoyable kick-around with a bunch of my old mates, always attempting to relive past glories, this afternoon turned out to be probably one of the most traumatic moments of my life. Twenty minutes into the game the opposition left full-back collapsed and had a cardiac arrest.

As a cardiologist I've managed hundreds of cardiac arrests in a hospital, with staff assisting me and all of the available equipment. Here I was, with another doctor, George Blackwood – a member of the

Defence Force – but with no equipment. Fortunately we were only a few kilometres away from one of Sydney's major teaching hospitals.

After I'd assessed that the man was in cardiac arrest, with no heartbeat and the cessation of respiration, we began cardiopulmonary resuscitation. Interestingly, over the last few years the medical profession has come to realise that mouth-to-mouth resuscitation is of no value in this situation. So therefore, alternating with George, I commenced cardiac massage. However, after five minutes or so, I felt that this man was probably not going to survive. We persisted, though, and while I think it took an ambulance somewhere between 10 and 15 minutes to arrive, who knows how fast time goes in that sort of situation?

When the ambulance arrived, we applied the paddles and electrodes, with the current applying a shock. I continued the cardiac massage and within about 30 seconds the man returned to a reasonably normal rhythm. He continued to take occasional breaths as well and once he established a reasonable rhythm his breathing returned. During the five-minute trip back to the Royal North Shore Hospital, he regained consciousness and chatted with the ambulance men.

As luck would have it, Professor Helge Rasmussen – a senior cardiologist at the hospital – was, at the time, performing angiograms on patients and rushed this man in to perform an urgent coronary angiogram. Three hours after his initial cardiac arrest, our patient was in having bypass surgery. Three days later, he rang to thank me for saving his life. Of course, credit also has to go to Dr George Blackwood.

Much less than 5 per cent of people who suffer out-of-hospital cardiac arrests survive, and many of these with a significant degree of brain damage. Also, had this man not had his cardiac arrest on a soccer field with two competent trained doctors, he would almost certainly have had his event at some time over the following few days. This could have been while he was sleeping, walking down the street, or potentially while driving; maybe even causing the death of other people as a consequence. So I feel very honoured to have had the skills and training to be able to help in this situation.

Managing hundreds of cardiac arrests in a hospital with staff and equipment is one thing, but using your bare hands with a successful outcome suggests there were greater forces at work in this particular case than pure human involvement. I'm not sure what those forces were but I'm glad they were helping me that day.

SCREENING

In an ideal world with no cost restraints, the least invasive, most accurate screening assessment should be offered to anyone at risk of the disease. This screening test should satisfy the following criteria:

- The underlying disease to be screened for has a long phase in which no symptoms are apparent. AVD fits this criterion.
- The screening test has general acceptance within the scientific community with trial data to support its use.
- By detecting the disease early, the quality and quantity of life will be positively altered.
- The interventions suggested based on the results of the screening test are safe and effective. The benefits of these interventions should outweigh the known long-term side effects of treatment.

The side effects should be considerably less than the consequences of not treating the disease.

- The procedures should be easily performed (including not time consuming) and inexpensive.
- The population screens should comply with the advice and the intervention suggested.
- The prevalence and seriousness of the disease justifies the cost of screening and treatment.
- The suggested treatment to prevent the manifestations of the disease is acceptable and effective.

It is my opinion that more sophisticated screening techniques should be offered to targeted groups. These groups should be based on age, sex and level of risk, based on standard risk factors.

The first step is to establish where you are at the moment:

Clinical assessment – the most important test any doctor can perform on a patient is to take a careful, thorough clinical history. It has been long said – and I totally agree – that a good, solid clinical history can diagnose well over 90 per cent of conditions and the medical tests used are purely there to confirm the diagnosis. One of the major problems of heart disease is that, in around 30 per cent of cases, the first sign of a heart attack is sudden death. This may be the case, but I'd suggest that almost everyone gets a warning that they usually ignore.

Basically, if you have any history of unexplained chest discomfort, from the tip of your nose down to your belly button – it doesn't have to be frank pain – you need to get it checked. Interestingly, only 5 per cent of chest pain is actually cardiac, but of course it is that 5 per cent that can lead you to drop dead in the street if it isn't detected. I have numerous patients coming to see me who say they have pain in their heart. Actually, they don't. They have pain in their chest that is not cardiac, but that is my decision, not theirs, and that's why you need to seek help when you have symptoms.

Symptoms aside, have you already had a heart problem? Have you suffered a heart attack, had coronary artery bypass or a stent inserted into your arteries? Do you suffer angina? (Angina is defined as pain in the chest which occurs with exertion or stress and which is eased by rest.) Have you had a coronary angiogram? (A dye study of your coronary arteries.)

The clinical history should be followed by a careful and thorough physical examination. I see some patients who tell me their overworked, time-poor local doctor doesn't even check their blood pressure, let alone perform a thorough examination.

The second aspect of an appropriate medical assessment is **blood testing**. I perform what I term advanced cardiac pathology, which involves the following blood tests:

1. Full lipid (blood fat) profile – cholesterol, HDL cholesterol, triglycerides, Apolipoprotein B/A1; Lipoprotein (a); LDL Subfractions (if available);
2. Blood sugar level;
3. Highly Sensitive C-reactive Protein (HsCRP) – a non-specific marker of inflammation;

4. Homocysteine – an indirect estimate of cell repair;
5. General tests – full blood count, electrolytes, kidney and liver function and uric acid, along with vitamin D levels.

(If you take a statin drug to lower your cholesterol, make sure that your doctor always collects a CPK level. This is a muscle enzyme that may be affected by statin therapy.)

A combination of all of the above tests gives additional information to your clinical assessment. I'd recommend these tests for all males over 40 and all females over 50 with a greater than 10 per cent, 10-year cardiovascular risk on a typical risk calculator mentioned previously.

Additional risk assessments

Arterial screening

The most important issue in cardiovascular risk assessment is not your cholesterol level or your family history but how much 'muck' (i.e. fat build-up and other substances) you have in your arterial wall.

A good, simple, non-invasive, totally painless method for assessing your arterial health is known as arterial screening. Basically, arterial screening measures arterial stiffness. The stiffer your arteries, the more fat you tend to have and thus the higher your risk. It's important to point out that no test in medicine is fail-safe, and the less invasive the test, usually the more chance the information obtained is not as robust as a more invasive test.

In cardiology, we view the coronary angiogram (dye study of the heart) as the gold standard for assessing heart disease. Although this is a great test, it is invasive. It involves a catheter being inserted into the femoral artery in the groin and then manoeuvred through the arterial system into the coronary arteries. Dye is then flushed through these arteries and any blockages are accurately detected. Although the risk of this test is very low, it does involve catheters travelling through the arterial system, a rather large dose of radiation, a visit to the hospital and a substantial cost to the individual and the health system.

Back to arterial screening. I believe this simple screening test should be offered to all people over the age of 35–40, and sooner if they have a higher risk (based on my previous comments).

Coronary calcium scoring

The best current method for determining the degree of coronary athero-sclerosis, however, and therefore coronary risk, is CT scanning of the coronary arteries, also known as coronary calcium scoring. Coronary calcium scoring provides an historical picture of your coronary arteries, which is a surrogate marker for the accumulation of fat in the arteries over the decades up to the point of scanning.

Here's the scoring ranking:

Zero – lowest cardiac risk. The predicted 10-year risk is only 1 per cent, which is much less than the majority of the population;
1–10: trivial calcification;
10–100: mild calcification;
100–400: moderate calcification;
greater than 400: severe calcification.

A calcium score higher than 400 predicts a 50 per cent 10-year risk, which makes it a much stronger risk predictor than cholesterol levels, blood pressure, diabetes and cigarette smoking. The calcium itself is not the problem. In fact, calcium is used by the body as a strengthening agent. The commonest site for calcium is, of course, in the bones, to make the bones stronger.

If the body detects an area of weakness, such as fat build-up in the wall of the artery, it will send in calcium to act as a scaffold to make the artery stronger, so it won't break down. Unfortunately, if you continue to bombard your arteries with modern living, the fat continues to build up in the wall and thus the calcium builds up attempting to stabilise the fat. Calcium is very easily seen by a CT scanner and therefore is a very good marker for the degree of fat you have in your arteries.

Let me also make the point that calcium in the arteries has nothing to do with the calcium you take in your diet or in supplement form. In fact, there is now a very strong link between low vitamin D levels (which is a very important controller of calcium metabolism) and a higher risk for heart disease.

Coronary calcium scoring is low-dose radiation, usually around four to five chest x-rays' worth, and relatively inexpensive. It doesn't require any injections and its results are very reproducible.

I should make a comment as well about virtual angiography, otherwise known as intravenous coronary angiography. This also uses a CT scanner but is not the same as coronary calcium scoring. It does involve an intravenous injection with dye and there is also a considerable amount of radiation involved with this technique. It is my strong opinion that it should not be used as a screening test for heart disease, although it does have other utilities.

I believe that the majority of people should consider having a coronary calcium score at some stage in their middle age. For men, I'd suggest somewhere between 45 and 50 years old, for women 55 to 60 years.

The reason for the age difference is that women tend to lag 10 years behind men in their coronary risk. This is usually because of the hormonal protection afforded by oestrogen and progesterone. When women begin menopause, their risk for heart disease significantly increases.

Stress tests are no indication

I would like to comment about executive stress testing and the new risk clinics that have sprung up all over the world, offering stress testing as a form of screening for heart disease. Very occasionally, a basic stress test will pick up someone with severe disease who has no symptoms, and examples like this are lauded in front of the media as being strong justification to take this test. Usually there are print, radio and, at times, television commercials encouraging this fear in people.

As I've mentioned, the first presentation of heart disease in 30 per cent of cases is sudden death, and if I thought basic exercise testing could prevent this carnage, I would also be a strong supporter of these techniques. The problem is that the thinking behind this is seriously flawed.

Although stress testing is easy to perform and relatively inexpensive, it is not a predictor of future risk. The reason for this is that an exercise test is basically looking for reduced blood flow from blockages in arteries. Atherosclerosis occurs in the wall, with the channel where the blood flows being open – in the majority of cases – until the very last minute, before the person either dies suddenly or has a major heart attack. Thus, it is only techniques that look at the wall that are truly predictive. The only non-invasive tests that examine the arterial wall are arterial screening, coronary calcium scoring and carotid ultrasound.

Even coronary angiography only looks at the channel and does not examine the wall, and we now know that there are numerous people with very severe atherosclerosis who have normal to near normal coronary angiograms. So, coronary angiography should not be seen as a screening test for heart disease either.

CHAPTER 3

More modern killers

Cancer

After heart disease, number two on the killer hit parade is the big C. In the 1920s, cancer killed only 3 per cent of the population. The latest figures see it taking off at somewhere between 30 and 35 per cent. Some health pundits predict that cancer may surpass cardiovascular disease as the numero uno killer over the next few decades. Is this bad luck or is there a good reason for the increasing rate of this very tragic condition?

Firstly, and most obviously, we're living longer. Our cells don't repair themselves as efficiently and we lose the normal elasticity of youth, not just in our skin (as seen by the increasing number of wrinkles that start spreading over the age of 50), but also our organs, muscles and joints stiffen up as well, for the same reason.

As well, the longer we live, the more mutations (or abnormal, potentially cancer-producing changes) occur in our DNA. The combination of living for decades past our use-by date of 30 to 40 years, and our increasing exposure to various synthetic chemicals, radiation and chronic stresses overwhelms our normal cell repair. Years of this exposure causes these mutations to occur.

Health care

You may be somewhat shocked when I tell you that coming in at number three, with its head placed firmly between its knees, is Western health care. Each year, in the USA alone, there are over 100,000 deaths from the appropriate prescription of medications.

I'm not even counting overdoses, inappropriate therapy or wrongly administered treatments here, i.e. mistakes by doctors, nurses or pharmacists. I'm actually referring to side effects which occur through sheer bad luck. Such side effects can be anything from a life-ending allergic reaction to depletion of the body's electrolytes by diuretics leading to a cardiac arrest. There are a group of drugs in cardiology known as anti-arrhythmics used for people with disorders of heart rhythms. Unfortunately, in some cases, they can induce what is termed a pro-arrhythmia, which basically induces a worse rhythm disturbance than you had in the first place. A recent study from the USA has suggested that two thirds of medication-related admissions to hospital in people over the age of 65 were due either to blood-thinning drugs used typically in people with cardiovascular disease or reactions to diabetic treatments.

I'm not against drugs, nor am I a 'basher' of the pharmaceutical industry. Strong medicine has strong effects, but in certain cases, it also has strong side effects. The appropriate use of pharmaceutical therapy has saved many lives, but has also ended a few as well. If you read the long list of potential side effects in the package insert that comes with all pharmaceuticals, you would never take a drug.

Drugs aside (I'll deal with them in much greater detail later), we're still left with the complications of medical procedures and operations.

Even in the most skilled hands, things go wrong. Operations can be complicated by wound infections, bleeding, post-operative pneumonia, kidney failure, bed sores – and the list goes on. There is also the major, ever-present and increasing problem of super-bugs. Golden staph (known as MRSA), VRE (Vancomycin-resistant Enterococcus) and *Clostridium difficile* are now major issues in hospitals throughout the world.

Serious medical conditions need to be treated but this may come at a significant price. Typically, when a person develops a serious illness, it's at a time in their life when they're either very stressed and/or their immunity is down. If this illness takes them into a hospital, it doesn't require much for one of the super-bugs to set up shop somewhere in their body. Mind you, it's very important to realise that if the initial condition that took them into hospital in the first place wasn't treated, it would possibly also lead to their death and not be seen as a medical complication leading to death. In many ways, this is a bit like rearranging the deck chairs on the *Titanic*.

Dementia

An increasing problem in the modern world is dementia in all its forms. All people with Alzheimer's disease have dementia, but not all dementia is caused by Alzheimer's. Alzheimer's is a specific dementing illness – with no definite cause – which affects a significant proportion of the population as they age. By age 85, it affects one in five women and one in 10 men. It starts with memory loss and slowly progresses to an inability to cope with the normal activities of daily living.

Lung disease

Chronic lung disease, either in the form of cigarette-related emphysema, chronic bronchitis or the very common condition of asthma, is another major cause of death in the modern world. There are a number of less common conditions such as bronchiectasis, which is damage to segments or, at times, even the entire lung by a variety of severe infections or genetic lung disorders, the most common and well known being cystic fibrosis. Another well publicised but not overly common group of chronic lung diseases are the occupational lung disorders, the top of the pops here being asbestosis. Once you're diagnosed with one of these conditions, you should be under the care of an expert respiratory physician.

Osteoporosis

You may be surprised to read that osteoporosis is a common killer these days. Osteoporosis is defined as the progressive loss of bone mineral such as calcium, leading to fragile and brittle bones. A fracture, especially of the lower limbs or the spine, can leave you immobile and thus more prone to infections from pneumonia, bed sores or urinary tract infections, along with an increasing tendency to develop deep vein thrombosis. If a large clot in the deep veins in your legs breaks away, it might travel into your lungs, leading to a pulmonary embolus. At times, this can be lethal.

Auto-immune diseases

Also potentially deadly are a whole host of disorders known as auto-immune diseases. The most common is rheumatoid arthritis, followed by a number of thyroid diseases and the rather common condition lupus.

The common theme here is the body's immune system turning against itself. This auto-immune reaction sets up inflammation in different organs, depending on the particular types of antibodies formed. Although medical science isn't 100 per cent sure of the actual cause, it is believed that in genetically predisposed individuals, certain toxins such as viruses and other infections set off this abnormal immune reaction in the body, leading to these diseases.

While there are no known cures, in the vast majority of cases there are a number of highly effective pharmaceutical therapies that are available to control auto-immune diseases. As with all diseases, an accurate diagnosis is the first step – this typically requires a thorough evaluation by a specialist in that particular field of medicine.

Infections

Although the field of microbiology and infectious diseases has advanced to extraordinary levels of understanding and treatment, people are still dying from infections. Viruses such as HIV, herpes and hepatitis, not to mention the devastating Ebola and Marburg viruses, are still taking people off the planet.

If you throw third world countries into the mix, infections are the second commonest cause of disease, after cardiovascular disease. Malaria and tuberculosis are still major killers in these areas, despite the availability of effective treatments. These don't always reach those who need them most.

Addictive illnesses

Tragically, addictive illnesses are also responsible for a significant number of deaths. Humanity has discovered many destructive methods of addiction and the commonest cause of addiction-related death in our society is cigarette smoking. This accounts for around 80 per cent of addiction-related deaths. There are an estimated one billion smokers on the planet and recent figures suggest that over 600,000 deaths per year worldwide are due to passive cigarette smoking.

Seventeen per cent of addiction-related deaths are related to alcohol abuse and 3 per cent are due to illegal drugs. Why is this figure so low, you may ask? Because the stuff is harder to get and more expensive. Unfortunately, the studies clearly show that rates of addiction, drug abuse, binge drinking and cigarette use are clearly related to cost and availability.

In Australia alone, the Federal Government reaps around $3 billion per year from the tax excise on cigarettes. It pays around $8 billion per year due to the diseases created by cigarettes, but saves enormous amounts of money on paying out pensions because smokers die on average 10 to 15 years earlier than anyone else. So, keep puffing, all you cigarette smokers, you're doing your bit for the country!

Suicide

A very unfortunate but ever-present statistic are the ongoing deaths from accidents, murder and suicide. The major point I'd like to make here is that suicide is almost always related to the very common disorder of brain chemicals known as endogenous depression.

If something bad happens in your life, such as the death of a loved one, and you feel depressed, you're not suffering endogenous depression – you're suffering grief, a sense of loss.

Endogenous depression is a completely different condition that may be related to a significant life trauma, but equally can occur for no reason. Also, endogenous depression is strongly associated with physical illnesses. Forty per cent of patients undergoing coronary artery bypass graftings suffer a temporary (usually) depressive illness.

Endogenous depression is thought to be due to reductions in the brain chemical serotonin. Once these brain chemicals are reduced to a critical level, you feel life isn't worth living and thus may attempt to commit suicide, or even be successful. This is precisely why you should seek help if you have any combination of these underlying symptoms:

1. fatigue;
2. early morning wakening (you wake at two or three in the morning and can't get back to sleep for an hour or two);
3. feeling of depression/loss of interest/sense of hopelessness.

Finally, there are a number of other illnesses that deserve a mention, such as chronic kidney and liver disorders. An exhaustive list is certainly not within the scope or spirit of this book, but I believe it's important to understand the potential issues that may arise at some stage in your life and also to give some insight into why hospitals are continually chock-a-block with patients.

For some of these modern killers, I'll highlight specific tips within the following categories:

1. *Take the test*

   Within each disease category, modern medicine has developed very accurate screening, diagnostic and monitoring tools to allow modern health professionals to manage disease risk assessment and target a treatment.

2. *Lifestyle factors*

   I'm always disturbed when a patient arrives in my office with the delusion that his or her drug therapy or vitamins are the answers to their health issues. Michael, a patient of mine for around a decade, is a good example. He has undergone a coronary bypass procedure and has since required a couple of coronary stents. He is diabetic and hypertensive and recently came to my office and plonked around 20 vitamins on my desk, along with six pharmaceutical agents. His plan was to discuss with me the appropriate use of all of these various therapies.

   The problem was the elephant in the room that Michael was avoiding. The elephant was, in fact, Michael himself – he was grossly overweight. He was prepared to spend his meagre income on drug and natural therapies, but didn't seem prepared to put the effort into where it was most important – melting away his gut.

3. *Targeted supplementation*

Vitamins and other forms of nutraceutical therapies are termed supplements. What are they supplements to? A healthy lifestyle. You'd be shocked by the number of patients I have managed over the years – like Michael – who are obese or smoke, but still swallow a bucket of vitamins on a daily basis. Supplements only work if the basic substance of your life, i.e. your lifestyle habits, is healthy and lifelong.

I'll demonstrate how vitamins are only about 5 to 10 per cent of the answer, as opposed to the 70 per cent contribution from lifestyle, and they only tend to work over a long period of time. Also, there is no one-size-fits-all approach. Not everyone benefits from vitamins, just as not everyone benefits from pharmaceutical therapy. As medicine advances, we are providing better methods for targeting who will benefit from certain types of foods, supplements and drugs.

4. *Orthodox medicine works*

I'm always bemused by patients of mine who are very resistant to taking any form of pharmaceutical therapy or are very suspicious of the relationship between orthodox doctors and pharmaceutical companies.

Strong medicine has strong side effects, but it's also very important to realise that it has strong benefits as well. The last 50 years have seen tremendous advances in medical and surgical therapies. There is no doubt we don't have all the answers, but there is also no doubt that modern medicine saves many more lives than it harms.

As one example, in the 1960s and '70s the death rate from heart attack once you'd made it to hospital was around 30 per cent. Now it has dropped to 2 to 3 per cent. This has nothing to do with improved lifestyles or complementary medicines – this is the raw power of modern medical therapies and techniques.

When I ask a patient why they don't want to take a pharmaceutical therapy, the typical answer is that they don't like putting unnatural chemicals into their bodies.

My retort to this is: have you eaten today? Did you use deodorant? Have you breathed the air in any large city? We live in a synthetic world where it's impossible to avoid synthetic chemicals.

Also, just because something is natural doesn't make it harmless. A snake bite can kill you rather rapidly without the appropriate anti-venom. Many people have very severe allergic responses to very natural chemicals.

5. *Follow-up*

There's no doubt that we all need a strong, long-term relationship with a trusted health professional who will organise appropriate preventative health strategies over a number of years. Regular contact and management with your doctor is a vital part of the management of all diseases.

CARDIOVASCULAR DISEASE

1. *Take the test*

    For most people without a family history of rampant heart disease, I see age 40 as a good time to start your cardiovascular surveillance. Take the simple test below, and if you tick any of these boxes I'd suggest you start at age 30.

    a. **Do you have a high cholesterol – or any type of abnormal fat profile – in the blood?**

        A number of people below age 40 have not had their cholesterols checked, so age 40 is a good time to start. If you're going to have that initial blood test, it may be advisable to have the more extensive advanced cardiac panel (ACP).

    b. **Do you have high blood pressure?**

        It's my firm opinion that any time a person over the age of 30 visits a doctor, regardless of the reason, their blood pressure should be checked. It takes 30 seconds for the doctor to stand up, put the cuff on your arm and take a reading. If you're over the age of 50, high blood pressure is by far the most important cardiovascular risk factor – much more so than cholesterol. I'm not saying cholesterol is unimportant, but the value of total cholesterol (not the more intricate breakdown I am suggesting with the advanced cardiac panel) is overemphasised by both the medical profession and the public. On the other hand, I believe the vital importance of maintaining a healthy blood pressure is understated and needs more attention and publicity than cholesterol appears to receive.

c. **Are you a previous or current smoker?**

It's also important to estimate your cumulative risk, so the two additional important questions here are length of time smoked (years) and number of cigarettes smoked per day (average). The good news is that after two years of giving up smoking, your risk for cardiovascular disease falls closer to that of a non-smoker. The bad news is that the same is not true for lung cancer or chronic lung disease.

d. **Are you a diabetic (or even pre-diabetic)?**

As most people are aware, there are two common types of diabetes, termed type 1 and type 2. (Can you imagine the millions of dollars paid to the think tank that came up with that classification!) Although not always the case, it is simple and reasonable to consider type 1 diabetes as the condition typically affecting children aged two to 12.

The pancreas, which sits behind the stomach, has a number of functions but is best known as the site of insulin production. Insulin is the major hormone in glucose (or sugar) metabolism and regulation. In type 1 diabetes, the pancreas fails, and if undetected the person develops a life-threatening condition known as diabetic ketoacidosis, with a marked rise in blood sugar, a serious aberration in blood chemistry known as metabolic acidosis, and without appropriate treatment – including insulin therapy – a progression to coma and death.

The initial presentation of this condition is marked fatigue, excessive thirst and passing excessive urine. Sufferers of type 1 diabetes are dependent on insulin administered by injections anywhere between one to five times per day, to achieve reasonable control of their blood sugar. Insulin may also be administered via a pump. Researchers are working on nasal insulin, along with pancreatic and islet cell transplants, but I believe the next major step in this regard will be stem cell therapy.

The much more common form of diabetes is type 2 (around 90 per cent). This type has a much stronger genetic inheritance. If one of your parents is a type 2 diabetic, you have around a 50 per cent chance of developing the condition. The gene for type 2 diabetes is even more common than this. In chapter one, I mentioned the insulin resistance genes. These are the pre-cursors to type 2 diabetes. With 30 per cent of Caucasians, 50 per cent of Asians and close to 100 per cent of people with varying shades of dark skin having the gene for insulin resistance, it is not surprising type 2 diabetes is very common. Around 10 per cent of the Australian population is a type 2 diabetic.

From the above figures, it will come as no surprise that type 2 diabetes is a major issue in Australian Aborigines and Torres Strait Islanders. The insulin resistant gene is a great advantage as a hunter-gatherer, but is exactly the opposite in the modern world.

e. **Do you have any family members who started their cardiac career before age 60?**

If you were foolish enough to pick the wrong relatives (and many of us were, in more ways than one), your risk for cardiovascular disease is significantly increased. For example, if your father suffered a heart attack at age 52, I wouldn't wait until age 40 to have your first preventative assessment. I'd start at 30. If your mother had a heart attack before menopause, I'd have that assessment at around the age of 25 or even earlier (depending on the medical history).

Tim's story

Tim was 28 years old. He was a high flyer with everything to live for. He'd started his own very successful financial business a few years before and was rapidly accumulating wealth. He drove fast cars, enjoyed the company of beautiful young women, smoked cigarettes and, at times, engaged in substance abuse.

But Tim had also picked the wrong relatives. His mother had an extremely high cholesterol level despite the fact that she wasn't particularly overweight and lived a rather moderate lifestyle. His father had coronary artery bypass grafting in his 50s, which was blamed on his very stressful lifestyle.

Tim had inherited his mother's cholesterol abnormality, known as familial hypercholesterolemia. (This name was obviously invented by the same think-tank that named type 1 and type 2 diabetes.) Although Tim's mother had no history of cardiovascular disease, the combination of this inherited high cholesterol, his father's history of premature cardiovascular disease and Tim's excessive lifestyle all contributed to Tim's early demise. He tried the statin drugs but didn't like the side effects, so he stopped the treatment without discussing this with his doctor. This turned out to be a fatal mistake.

He was holidaying with friends in Bali and collapsed in the surf. Attempts were made to resuscitate him, but these failed. So a 28-year-old man with everything to live for had met an early demise.

Tim knew he had a problem, but chose to ignore it. You may not realise you have a problem, but, hopefully, reading this book will inspire you to take action. Although many people are given the genetic short straw, these days modern medicine has many effective therapies that can minimise the damaging effects of these genetics.

Regarding the appropriate lifestyle modification, targeted supplementation and the use of orthodox medicine, I will detail all of these later in the book.

CANCER

1. *Take the test*

   The risk of being diagnosed with cancer before age 75 is about one in three for males and one in four for females. If you extend this to 85 years of age, it's about one in two for males and one in three for females.

   In Australia, the most common cancers reported were: prostate – 19,403 cases; bowel – 14,234 cases; breast – 12,670 cases; melanoma – 10,342 cases; lung – 9,703 cases. These five cancers accounted for around 61 per cent of all cancer diagnoses.

i. **Prostate cancer**

Screening for this very common cancer is extremely contentious. To give you some important figures regarding this disease, see www.prostate.org.au.

A chance for diagnoses for prostate cancer: men in their 40s – one in 1000; men in their 50s – 12 in 1000; men in their 60s – 45 in 1000; men in their 70s – 80 in 1000. Each year, around 3300 men in Australia die from prostate cancer. Close to 20,000 new cases are diagnosed each year. One in nine men in Australia develop prostate cancer in their lifetime.

The problem with screening for prostate cancer is not its accuracy, but rather the disease itself. Screening for prostate cancer has left the medical community divided because the disease is so variable. It has been stated that if you perform a careful autopsy on every man over the age of 80, to some extent you will find prostate cancer in virtually everyone.

In some men, prostate cancer will be an aggressive disease that spreads early and may lead to premature death. In others, it has a less aggressive course and with appropriate early therapy it may be cured. But there is another group of men who will take the disease with them to their grave, because all it did was hang around in the prostate playing poker with a few of its prostatic mates in one of the seedier lobes, but it couldn't be bothered contacting the travel agent to organise a trip to the local lymph nodes or more distant organs.

Thus, prostate cancer is not all things to all people and this is precisely the problem. Detecting early prostate cancer in many people puts them on the road to invasive investigations and even more invasive treatments that they may not have needed in the first place. But in other people, if the disease is not detected early, you may be taken off this planet at far too young an age.

The other big problem here is that the initial tests we have are not that great at deciding which category you're in. It is, however, recommended that you start your prostate screening at age 50. If you have a family history of prostate cancer in either your brother, father or grandfather, you should start at 40.

It's important to note that the symptoms of prostate cancer may occur quite late, but if you have any of the following you should see a doctor immediately:

- Waking frequently at night to urinate
- Sudden or urgent need to urinate
- Difficulty in starting to urinate
- Slow flow of urine and difficulty in stopping
- Discomfort when urinating
- Painful ejaculation
- Blood in the urine or semen
- Decrease in libido
- Reduced ability to achieve an erection

If you're interested in more information, I'd strongly suggest you go to the excellent website www.prostate.org.au, the website of the Prostate Cancer Foundation of Australia.

The initial screening for prostate cancer is a digital rectal examination, otherwise known as a DRE, along with a PSA, which stands for prostate specific antigen blood test. I'd venture to say that the vast majority of men don't put the digital rectal examination in the top 10 of their most enjoyable experiences. I'd also venture to say (despite being a card-carrying member of the male union) that men are a bunch of wimps. Ladies, can you imagine a male having a baby? It wouldn't happen, for more reasons than pure biology.

Recently, from Surrey in the south of England, a new urine test has been developed known as EN2, or engrailed-2. This EN2 is much more specific for prostate cancer, detecting 60 to 70 per cent of prostate cancers with a very low false positive rate, unlike the PSA test which has a false positive rate of around 50 per cent.

The DRE is the most accurate method currently available for early detection of prostate cancer. The PSA remains a very contentious issue. I've heard some authorities state that they'd sue a doctor who performed a PSA on them. The problem with the PSA is that it is too sensitive. If, for example, you have a digital rectal examination and then a PSA within the next few days, the DRE itself can increase the PSA, giving you a false reading.

PSA can also vary with sexual activity. If you haven't emptied your prostate for a week or so and then have the PSA checked, this may slightly elevate your PSA level as well. Certainly, a prostate infection may put your PSA through the roof.

At times, a PSA is performed – without the DRE – sparking major concern. It is my suggestion that, when you turn 50, have the DRE, wait a few weeks, and then have the PSA as part of your comprehensive check-up, which should also include the advanced cardiac panel.

If you get to the point where the DRE is abnormal and/or your PSA is high, (especially if you've had a few progressively rising levels), I'd suggest you seek a few opinions from well-respected urologists. This, more than any other cancer, is an area where you need to make a very informed decision. Search the internet for information and opinions, but listen to the experts and decide for yourself who appears to be making the most compelling case.

Cyberchondria

Seeing as I've just encouraged you to search the net for information, at this point I'd like to bring in the new concept of cyberchondria. A recent survey revealed that around 60 per cent of Americans use the internet for health advice. Around one third of those surveyed stated that they changed their mind about how their condition should be treated after surfing the net; this is despite the fact that there is growing evidence that much of the web-based information is unreliable.

You'll draw some comfort in knowing that Wikipedia – a commonly used site for information – has been independently studied and most experts agree that it is very accurate. One major problem, however, is that some pharmaceutical companies have been known to remove negative information about their drugs.

Some of the more reliable medical information sites are:

Medlineplus: www.medlineplus.gov – from the US National Library of Medicine;

NHS: www.nhs.uk – from the UK National Health Service;

Mayo Clinic – www.mayoclinic.com;

Web MD – www.webmd.com: written by doctors and reviewed by an independent board.

ii. Bowel Cancer

This cancer is very personal for me as both my parents suffered from this condition. Therefore my chance of developing bowel cancer is close to 100 per cent, unless of course I take the test. Because 80 Australians die each week from bowel cancer, it's important to be vigilant. So, what is the test for bowel cancer?

The most simple test is known as faecal occult blood investigation. It is a simple, easy-to-perform test. In Australia, the National Bowel Cancer Screening program offers testing to all people turning 50, 55 or 65.

In Australia, the above people are sent invitations and kits in the mail. You can perform the test in the privacy of your own home and then mail the kits to the designated pathology company. The tests are said to be around 80 per cent accurate.

Colonoscopy

The most accurate test for bowel cancer screening is definitely a colonoscopy. This is said to have a 96 per cent accuracy rate. I'd suggest that all people 50 years or older should have at least one colonoscopy in their lifetime. (And some people I know should have one a week without the anaesthetic!)

A colonoscopy is a long black tube known as an endoscope, which is placed in the rectum and views the entire colon, with the patient under sedation. It visualises the entire colon, detecting pre-cancerous lumps known as polyps, as well as established cancers.

If you have a family history of relatives suffering bowel cancer before age 65, you should start having colonoscopies at age 40, and consult your gastroenterologist as to how regularly you need to have them thereafter. This depends on the initial findings on the colonoscope.

Although none of this stuff sounds pleasant, I can assure you it is far more pleasant than dying from bowel cancer that is totally preventable if detected as a pre-cancerous polyp or a very early cancer.

iii. Breast Cancer

The risk of a woman developing breast cancer before the age of 75 is one in 11. The Breast Screening Australia program suggests women between the age of 50 and 70 have mammography every two years. There is a reasonable concern amongst women regarding the radiation dose, but as x-ray technology improves, the radiation is minimal despite maintaining good quality screening.

There is still, however, ongoing debate as to whether the radiation from mammograms induces more cancers than it detects. Most experts in the area dispute this concern and claim the studies strongly suggest the value of screening mammography.

Some alternative practitioners push the benefits of a technique known as thermography. The vast majority of orthodox doctors do not believe there is enough evidence for this to be an acceptable replacement for mammography.

Breast self-examination should be encouraged on a regular basis in all women. (And I know a number of males who would be happy to participate in this program.) Speaking of males, although it is rare, they can also suffer from breast cancer. When a male develops breast cancer, he is usually a carrier of the BRCA1 or 2 gene – the common genetic cause of breast cancer in women. So, males with a very strong family history of breast cancer in their female relatives should be aware of this possibility.

Regardless, no-one disputes that early detection of breast cancer gives you the best chance of cure.

iv. **Melanoma**

This is the worst type of skin cancer, and like almost all skin cancers, it is directly related to sun exposure. There are no screening tests apart from a thorough skin inspection by an expert in this area. Melanomas can occur anywhere on the skin, even in areas not particularly exposed to the sun. In rare cases, they can even occur in the retina.

v. **Lung Cancer**

There are not too many people who aren't aware of the link between cigarettes and lung cancer. Screening chest x-rays has not been shown to be of any value. However, a recent study showed that a screening lung CT scan in current or former smokers can reduce lung cancer deaths by around 20 per cent. Although non-smokers may develop lung cancer, there is no proven benefit for screening in this group.

Also, using nano technology via a breath test, a recent study from Israel demonstrated an accurate method to determine the early genetic changes associated with lung cancer.

2. *Lifestyle factors*

There are a number of lifestyle issues that may reduce your risk, as well as poor lifestyle choices that may do the opposite. Many are so obvious that they really don't deserve a mention, but purely for pig-headed people who don't appear to have got the message yet, I'll repeat them.

The obvious list for those people who believe it won't happen to them:

i. Don't smoke. And in case you missed it – don't smoke. It's not just lung cancer, but also blood, upper respiratory and esophageal cancers, to name the more common associations.

ii. Don't consume excessive amounts of alcohol – again, it's not just cirrhosis of the liver, but upper gastrointestinal cancers and, in pre-disposed individuals, liver cancer.

iii. Don't sunbake. We all know the dangers of excessive sun exposure, so why do you do it?

iv. Avoid exposure to toxic chemicals.

v. Don't live near nuclear power plants with faulty reactors.

Here are some specific, less well-known lifestyle tips for cancer prevention. Firstly, and very importantly, *use the organ for what it was designed for*. To give the most obvious example, you have these organs in your chest called your lungs. They were not designed for you to put a white stick in your mouth, light the end and then suck smoke into them. They are actually designed for breathing.

But this doesn't just apply to smoking. Let's go through the common cancers I've covered so far:

1. **Prostate** – the prostate was designed to be emptied on a regular basis. One of the reasons older men develop prostate cancer is related to the decreased regularity of prostatic emptying. To put this in less subtle terms: how many times a male ejaculates per week.

If you are rating yourself on a monthly basis, then you're already behind the eight ball (so to speak). For those of you who are unaware, sperm is produced in your testicles, but the delivery fluid of sperm – semen – is made in the prostate gland. I won't go into the complicated network of tubing that leads to the final result; suffice to say, my advice is to empty your prostate on a regular basis.

2. **Bowel** – here's an obvious one. Although this is not as 'in your face' as smoking, you should be using your gastrointestinal tract for what it was designed for. The function of the lower – or large – intestine, otherwise known as the colon (we have a variety of names for the organs of our body, purely to keep you confused – it maintains the magic and makes doctors seem a lot more intelligent than we really are!), is basically to form the final product that becomes your bowel action, stool, faeces (there go those names again).

Whatever you put in your mouth has three choices. It has to be absorbed into the body as part of our nutrient (and unfortunately quite often toxin) intake where it comes out the way it came in, i.e. you either spit it out or more dramatically vomit it out (don't you just hate throwing up?).

The third choice is out through the anus in the form of faeces. The colon was designed purely to remove natural substances from the natural environment of a hunter-gatherer. It wasn't designed to have to cope with all this processed, packaged rubbish masquerading as food, laden with synthetic fats, processed carbohydrates, excessive salt, preservatives and colourings, as well as a number of other additives given a variety of numbers that the vast majority of us couldn't be bothered to Google to find out what laboratory animal has developed which tumour when exposed to this stuff.

Also, here's a more specific form of colonic abuse you should incorporate into your anti-cancer armamentarium. Your colon really doesn't like being bombarded with nitrosamines from chargrilled steaks. Yes, those of you who feel it is your God-given right to cremate your steaks to blacker than the ace of spades should think again. If you enjoy that time-honoured tradition of the barbecue, make sure you're at the front of the line when the steaks are being handed out. The medium-rare recipients will have colons that will bless you forever.

Overall, the simple point I'm making here is to present your gastrointestinal tract with as much natural food as possible and also don't overload the poor thing.

3. **Breast** – for any males reading this, you may be shocked to realise that the breasts were not purely designed for our enjoyment; strangely, they were designed to feed babies. Over the years, there have been numerous studies relating the length of time between the onset of puberty in females and the first pregnancy. Another medically disturbing feature of our modern world is women delaying having babies. To make what will be the first of hopefully many politically incorrect comments, from a purely physiological

viewpoint the ideal time for a woman to have a baby is between 15 and 25 years old. Not only are the eggs at their prime, the breasts sit up and wait to hear the news that they're about to be given their big start.

Can you imagine the disappointment to those mammary glands eking out their existence on the front of the chest wall, just hoping for their big chance to strut their stuff, month in month out, but nothing happens? Unfortunately, for reasons I'll reinforce in later chapters, the rates of breast cancer have doubled over the past 20 or 30 years, especially during pregnancy.

4. **Melanoma** – I've already given this tip: don't sunbake. Slip, slop, slap. Use a hat, a beach umbrella and avoid the sun between the main burning times of 11 am to 4 pm. You need some vitamin D (the main source being the sun), but not too much. Here comes the balance theme again.

5. **Lung** – have I mentioned smoking?

3. *Targeted Supplements*

Multivitamins

There has been no convincing evidence that multivitamins do harm in regard to cancer. Many trials of multivitamins suggest a benefit, although this is still an area of controversy in the scientific world.

If you ask most orthodox doctors, they will rightly tell you that there is no good consistent evidence that any vitamins are of value, other than for people with a proven vitamin deficiency.

I agree. The clinical trial evidence just isn't there, but here's the problem.

Randomised Controlled Trials (RCTs)

Let me give you a quick – and hopefully not tedious – explanation for how these things work. RCTs are seen by orthodox science as the gold standard for the assessment for any drug, procedure or intervention. They are typically applied to drugs and usually are sponsored by a large pharmaceutical company that has the millions of dollars necessary to fund such large scale trials.

What usually happens is best explained by the following purely contrived scenario (the names have been changed to protect the not so innocent). A drug company, Pharma (how generic is that!), has developed (wait for it) a new drug. It has been in the planning and testing phase for 10 years, already at a cost of $500 million. This drug (let's call it Cholbust) is a totally new cholesterol-lowering agent that blocks a newly discovered pathway of cholesterol metabolism. It's been shown to be safe in a number of unsuspecting laboratory rats, who thought they were eating the usual delectable rat pellets so lovingly supplied by their handlers.

Their livers, kidneys, muscles and hearts continue to function and there were certainly fewer complaints of chest pain in the rats chewing on the Cholbust, but maybe the other rats were just a bunch of whingers with low pain thresholds.

So, let's move on to the RCT. Through a bunch of 'independent' academic researchers, Pharma screened around 50,000 subjects, weeding out around 40,000 because of what is known as exclusion criteria, i.e. significant pre-existing conditions such as cancer, kidney disease or severe end stage heart disease, or they didn't like their hair colour or their voting habits.

Pharma is now left with 10,000 ideal candidates (hardly representatives of a normal community), half of whom are given Cholbust for five years, the other half a sugar pill. At the end of the study period, the rates of heart attack, stroke, sudden death and a whole host of other factors are tested. Comparisons are then made between Cholbust and the sugar pill (or placebo) to see if Cholbust is a wonder drug or a rather expensive waste of Pharma's rather extensive cash base.

The results showed a 25 per cent reduction in the aforementioned events in the people taking the active pill. This all sounds very impressive, but when you hear a rather dramatic sounding reduction, it is important to realise that this is known as a relative reduction, not absolute reduction. So a 25 per cent reduction doesn't mean that of the 5000 on the treatment, there were 1250 fewer heart attacks, strokes or sudden deaths. It may only mean a reduction of 1 per cent down to .75 per cent which is also a 25 per cent reduction. When you do the numbers, this would be a reduction from 50 events to around 38 events, i.e. a reduction of 12 events – hardly earth shattering.

Pharma, however, wants you to assume that 25 per cent sounds a very substantial number. Often in these RCTs, the results are of this magnitude.

Once you are allocated either the active treatment or the placebo, you stay in that group for the final analysis. The big problem here is that a number of people in either group experience side effects or basically get sick of being in the study and therefore drop out.

One of the most disturbing and often quoted trials delivered a significant piece of nonsense as far as statistics are concerned. This trial was known as the Helsinki Heart Study, which studied the effects of an old-style cholesterol lowering pill, gemfibrozil, which is a fibrate drug. This group of drugs is very effective at lowering triglycerides, one of the fatty components.

One of the incidental findings from this trial was a statistically significant increase in the rate of murder and suicide in the active treatment group. Thus, we heard ridiculous statements in the media during the '90s when this trial was released, such as 'Heart pill increases the death rate from murder and suicide'.

When you actually read the true data, you realise what total and utter nonsense this is. The raw data is thus: in the few thousand allocated to the active treatment group, there were 10 deaths attributed to murder and suicide. In the placebo group there were only four deaths. But now here's the drum. Five of the 10 people in the active treatment group were not actually taking gemfibrozil at the time, as they had dropped out. Therefore, there were five deaths in the active group and nine deaths in those not taking gemfibrozil. Thus, gemfibrozil protects you against murder and suicide. Any sensible person can see what nonsense this is, but also how such low numbers, whether they are statistically significant or not, are really meaningless. The point I'm making is to be suspicious of any statistics you read.

Now, the point of this long diatribe is that it is my opinion that nutritional supplements should not be studied in the same fashion as their stronger, richer cousins, pharmaceutical drugs.

Supplements are not that strong, and in reality should be considered more like food than drugs. Although orthodox medicine looks at lifestyle in a totally different fashion (because it's hard to have a blinded placebo group when it comes to diet, exercise or stress relief), it is still more than happy to accept the results of the non-RCT analysis of these interventions.

In most cases it takes much longer for supplements to work than the typical five-year period used for drug trials. Now back to the multi-vitamin story. The longest trial in modern medicine reviewing a number of lifestyle habits, medication ingestion and vitamin use is the Nurses' Health Study. This has been going for around 30 years. Up to a period of 14 years, for the nurses who took multivitamins compared with those who didn't, there was no difference in cancer rates. However, when they analysed the data beyond 15 years there was a 75 per cent reduction in bowel cancer and a 25 per cent reduction in breast cancer. There are two important points here. Number one, the multivitamin had to contain at least 400 micrograms of folic acid to achieve the result. Number two, in women who consumed any alcohol at all, there was a slight but significant increase in the risk of breast cancer, unless they took the multivitamin with the 400 micrograms of folic acid.

Fruit and vegetables contain over 600 varying plant chemicals that have been shown in laboratory and experimental animals to have an inhibiting effect on cancers. The 10 per cent of the population who consume two to three pieces of fruit and three to five servings of vegeta-bles on a daily basis (one serving equals about half a carrot) have the lowest rates of cancer and heart disease.

Whether taking these chemicals and individually putting them in a pill or a capsule will treat or prevent cancer has never been proven. Many substances have been suggested as wonder pills, but I believe the evidence is just not there. There is probably some benefit in these substances, but it may not be that dramatic.

Among these suggested supplements have been Indole-3-Carbinol (one of the active ingredients in broccoli and other cruciferous vegetables), the anthocyanins (the substances that give purple and blue coloured fruits and vegetables their deep hue), and even a substance termed vitamin b17, a strange version of cyanide that appears to be toxic only to cancer cells, which occurs in apricot kernels, apple seeds, pomegranates and millet.

4. *Orthodox Medicine*

The appropriate use of surgical techniques, chemotherapy and radiotherapy have offered excellent longevity and, at times, reasonable palliation for a variety of cancers. The evidence base is certainly vast and growing.

Over the past 10 years there have been enormous advances in cancer therapy with marked improvement in targeted chemotherapy and radiotherapy. I'd strongly suggest that anyone diagnosed with cancer should see orthodox treatment as their mainstay. I believe the lifestyle interventions detailed previously are not negotiable. I also believe you should pursue the complementary techniques, which should be seen as a supplement to orthodox medicine.

5. *Follow-up*

Once you have any chronic illness, regular follow-up is vital. You must have regular assessments of your progress.

ALZHEIMER'S DISEASE AND OTHER FORMS OF DEMENTIA

1. *Take the test*

   If you have a family history of typical Alzheimer's disease, it's advisable to have:

   a. the apo E allele blood tests;

   b. the advanced cardiac panel (see Appendix), along with other additional tests – full blood count ESR, UEC, LFTs, calcium, phosphate;

   c. Imaging; Brain CT or MRI, carotid/vertebral dopplers (plus or minus CT coronaries, arterial screening);

   d. Neuropsychiatric testing, including a screen for depression

2. *Lifestyle factors*

   As I've described previously.

3. *Supplementation*

   Just imagine that the pharmaceutical world discovered a drug that could reduce progression to dementia by 50 per cent. There wouldn't be too many doctors who weren't bombarded by advertisements in medical journals and visits from drug reps and many academic professors would be flown around the world in the pointy end of the plane to discuss the extraordinary benefits of this particular drug.

   Well, recently a study was released showing just this very fact. There was a 50 per cent reduction in the progression of typical Alzheimer's-related changes on an MRI with a 12-month course of therapy. This information was relegated to a small column in one of the Australian medical magazines on around page 8, and no-one apart from me and the medical media actually discussed it at all. The reason is that the therapy used to reduce the progression of Alzheimer's disease by 50 per cent was, in fact, the combination of folic acid (800 micrograms daily), B6 (20 milligrams daily) and B12 (500 micrograms).

Regarding the use of supplementation with Alzheimer's disease, there have been a number of studies with varying and, at times, contradictory evidence regarding the benefits of supplementation for this devastating condition.

It is my opinion that the big problem with the trials for Alzheimer's disease is no different from all the other trials involving supplementation, i.e. too little, too late. The vast majority of these trials were in people with established, albeit mild, Alzheimer's disease.

Supplements with probable benefit (as a preventative), if used early for Alzheimer's disease:

i.   B group vitamins;

ii.   A combination of Brahmi (in varying preparations – phosphatidylserine 100 milligrams and Ginkgo biloba 3 grams);

iii. Vitamin E 500–1000 international units (combined with vitamin C 1000 milligrams);

iv.   Brain training – 'use it or lose it' is a vital principle when it comes to Alzheimer's disease prevention. It has long been known that there are a variety of techniques to maintain brain stimulation. It has been said for a number of years that regularly performing crosswords, Sudoku and other brain puzzles is a simple way to keep the brain active.

One recent study demonstrated five key factors in maintaining mental sharpness beyond the age of 70:

i. Maintain employment or an ongoing active interest in your field of endeavour;

ii. Stay involved in a variety of activities such as reading widely, travelling and avoiding dull routine;

iii. Be open to change;

iv. Be married or have a lifelong partner who is bright and optimistic;

v. Be optimistic yourself.

There's no doubt we'll be taken off the planet whether we like it or not (I can't imagine too many of us will actually like it!). Also, it is not easy to determine your disease of choice. But if you follow the principles set out in this book, you'll give yourself the best chance of delaying whatever your genes are driving you towards.

CHAPTER 4

ENERGY

How often do you hear someone say, 'I'm so tired I just can't function properly!' Fatigue, tiredness, lassitude – call it what you like – is a common epidemic of modern society. There are many different causes of lack of energy that I'll cover extensively in this chapter, but in many ways it can be traced back to the cellular level. So, before I cover the causes, let me give you an overview of the simple science.

We all know that oxygen is essential for the vast majority of life on earth. One simple way to end a person's existence is to cut off their oxygen supply. But do you know what oxygen is for? Why do we actually need it? Basically to react with glucose to form the unit of energy known as ATP. There are these magical structures within each cell called mitochondria where ATP is formed. Oxygen and glucose are the fuels that drive the production of ATP. As I've said previously, physiologically we were only designed to live 30 or 40 years, and once you've gone beyond your use-by date your energy-producing mechanisms don't work as well. The reason for this all comes down to mitochondrial DNA.

The dictionary definition of energy is the capacity for work or vigorous activity – a sense of vigour or power. But I suspect we all know what energy means when we feel we don't have it. You can lack physical energy, mental energy, emotional energy or even spiritual energy. But at times, we have boundless energy and feel like we could take on the world. So, I suppose a good working definition of energy is the act of performing tasks and functioning at the best of your ability. I think it's worth considering energy according to the five stages model:

1. *Body Health* – at the biochemical level I'd like to introduce the concept of the mitochondria. The mitochondria are the compartments of the cell that supply us with energy. We receive nutrients in two basic ways: (a) through our lungs in the form of oxygen; (b) through our gut in the form of macro- and micronutrients. The oxygen and the nutrients combine in a series of chemical reactions in the mitochondria that produce the unit of energy (the fuel for our cells – ATP, as I've mentioned). If you don't produce adequate and quality ATP, you lack energy.

   Without energy, the rather rapid consequence is your friends and loved ones attending your funeral.

   All of the metabolic pathways in the body are finely regulated and should not be abused. The body works in cycles, an obvious one being the 24 hour cycle. Over the eons we have evolved an energy system that is roughly divided into thirds. This is variable and certainly not the same for different people. You have around eight hours of active energy, eight hours of relaxation energy and eight hours where your body needs to sleep to replenish the energy you've spent during your waking hours. Although science is yet to unravel the mystery of sleep, try going without it and find out what lacking energy really means.

There are a number of theories of aging that I will elucidate in chapter six, but a major theory which achieved Professor Elizabeth Blackburn a Nobel Prize involves little caps at the end of your DNA called telomeres.

If you took one strand of DNA from any of your cells and unwound it in a straight line, it would be around two metres long. To overcome this issue (which would see us having to wear much bigger clothes) nature solved the problem by twisting and turning DNA into a rather tight but strangely well organised ball, so it could fit inside the nucleus of each cell (apart from the red cells which missed out in the nuclear department because haemoglobin kicked out the nucleus and took over early in the evolutionary stage).

At the ends of DNA are these small caps (telomeres) which are like the caps on the end of your shoelaces. Now here is the problem – DNA which was originally the same throughout the body was really only designed to last around 30 or 40 years as it initially adapted to the local conditions.

With each cell division, the DNA changes. The cells lining the gut turn over every four to five days. Skin cells are recycled every few weeks. Red cells last three to four months. The liver typically replaces itself every 300 to 500 days. The body is like any other structure on earth. It has a finite structure and a finite lifespan. It has its optimum function time and then it slowly (or at times rapidly) wears out.

With each cell division these little caps (the telomeres) shorten. There is an enzyme called telomerase which partially maintains the size of the telomeres and thus when disrupted may contribute to the ageing process, thus typically as we go beyond that enviable age of 40, our DNA has divided on so many occasions that it loses its vibrant ability to keep us looking, feeling and acting young. Unfortunately, a number of people continue to behave like juveniles all through their lives (despite how they look) but, for this chapter, let's stick to the mitochondria. Once your DNA has divided over a number of years, these mutations lead to reduced ATP synthesis.

So, is there anything you can do about this at a biochemical level? Well, the good news is yes. Elegant work spearheaded by Professor Tony Linnane and Frank Rosenfeldt in Melbourne has shown that taking high-dose coenzyme Q10 and magnesium orotate supplements bypasses these mutations in the mitochondrial DNA leading to the production of ATP, and thus increases energy levels.

Statin therapy: the biggest selling drug in the world is Atorvastatin (Lipitor), which is one of a number of statins used to lower cholesterol. All statins deplete coenzyme Q10 in the body. Around 10 per cent of people taking statins experience a degree of muscle aches and pains and/or stiffness, and a number of other people experience a degree of muscle weakness. Strangely, all the pharmaceutical-sponsored studies of statins (using only industry-approved, good quality, ideal patients) report just a 1 to 2 per cent incidence of muscle pain.

It is my strong opinion that all patients taking statin therapy should be taking supplements of coenzyme Q10 and magnesium orotate. I also strongly believe that all people over the age of 40 who would like extra energy (regardless of whether they do or do not take statins) should be taking the following every morning: coenzyme Q10 (300 mg) and magnesium orotate (400 mg).

2. *Environmental* – there is no doubt that your energy levels can be affected both by your micro and macro environment and I make a strong case for improving both these scenarios in the chapter on environmental health. Suffice to say there is no doubt that being in nature with fresh air is one example of a situation that can give you an energy boost.

3. *Genetic* – there is no doubt that we all have variable levels of energy. Some of this is genetically primed and in fact there are a number of (fortunately) rare diseases that affect the mitochondria and thus diminish energy reserves.

4. *Emotional* – with the 24-hour cycle I've mentioned, it won't shock you to read that if you have an issue in one of these eight hour blocks, you deplete your energy.

    Most of us work in some fashion. You may not have a paid job but there are still chores to be done, bills to pay etc. Once you've reached your active energy limit, you start to feel tired.

    Thus, the people who put in 12 hour days, six to seven days per week, will almost always burn themselves out in some way or other. I have some patients who say to me, 'Doc, I haven't had a holiday in 10 years,' and my reply is, 'Well, you're an idiot!' You're certainly living against your physiology if you don't actively manage your energy. If you'd like that premature heart attack, cancer or some obvious or not-so-obvious form of mental illness, keep stealing those extra hours of active energy on a daily basis and see what happens.

But it isn't just about those active eight hours: it's also about how you manage the other two blocks of eight hours. How do you spend your eight hours of relaxation energy? Do you arrive at home to a dysfunctional relationship? Do you spend your time overeating, drinking excess alcohol or involving yourself in other forms of addiction that aren't serving your true life purpose? Do you feel that sense of joy, peace and contentment with all aspects of your life?

When you're actively working, you don't have time to contemplate these vital aspects of your life. So, your allocated relaxing time should be spent on activities that instil this sense of joy, peace and contentment.

There's nothing wrong with enjoying a movie or watching your favourite TV show but it certainly doesn't serve you to spend hours sitting mindlessly in front of the television, not moving, apart from the 'toilet stop'. Typically, sitting in front of the television also involves consuming unnecessary comfort foods and often alcohol. This, combined with the inactivity, doesn't create a healthy environment and it certainly doesn't recharge your energy for the next day.

The third block is the sleeping block. In ancient times, sleep was seen as a vital aspect of life. Many tribes sat around after sleep, discussing the importance and meaning of dreams. We have a sleep cycle that occurs in five stages and we typically have four to five of these cycles per night. With each of these cycles, two of the phases are involved with deep sleep, which rejuvenates our body for the next day.

Without these repeating bouts of deep sleep, we cannot replenish our ATP stores in our cells and we don't function properly. My strong advice is to cultivate good sleeping habits.

I'd also strongly advise you to carefully manage all aspects of your energy. Don't overwork. See any stress as being like a garbage bin. If you don't empty the bin on a regular basis, the rubbish flows over the side and creates a horrible mess.

Thus, if you work hard, make sure the relaxation and sleep boxes of your 24-hour cycle are high quality and don't contribute to the depletion of your ATP.

5. *Mind Health* – this is the most profound aspect of energy management. If any aspect of your energy systems is disrupted, then, guess what, your energy is disrupted. In the second section of this book, I'll introduce the entire aspect of mind health. I will also introduce seven universal spiritual laws (I know it should be five, but who am I to argue with the universe?).

Protect your castle

As I've mentioned, I think you should see every cell in your body as an individual castle, which is either living in peace with the surrounding environment or at war and under attack. Each castle has its own inherent defence system and a number of allies it can call upon if an attack occurs.

The attacking army is our modern world and all its issues, including synthetic chemicals, excess intake of calories, excess electro-magnetic radiation, chronic life stresses, and disordered thinking and feeling. As we were not designed for this, any of these issues attack the cell and cause significant disruption. Each castle has a wall. If the castle has been well maintained, the wall is very sturdy. This wall is the major interface between the castle and the outside environment. If the outside environment is also peaceful, well maintained and its inhabitants are happy, living a balanced life, they'll interact well with the castle and its inhabitants. The environmental inhabitants will have robust and healthy trade with the castle and its occupants, with the cell and its surrounds being a contented healthy place. But if the surrounds of the castle are hostile, the castle is then in danger and all the energy the castle needs to defend itself is taken away from the energy the entire unit could be using to maintain its normal function.

I suspect you can see my point. Once you introduce unwanted assaults to the individual castles or the individual cells, the cells start to function poorly. A very good example here is one of the major poisons of modern society – trans fatty acids. TFAs are ubiquitous throughout modern processed packaged food, as well as a number of bakery items and one of our modern scourges, takeaway foods.

The main function of TFAs is to thicken and harden foods, so they can be kept inside a box or a container for months or even years. Unfortunately, these TFAs do the same things to your cell membranes. Being 75 per cent fat, these membranes (i.e. your castle walls) cannot discern between a healthy natural fat and a synthetic fat. The natural fats make the membrane fluid and flexible, allowing the normal flow of nutrients, natural chemicals and other cellular messengers into and out of the cell. The TFAs, however, make these membranes brittle and prone to crumbling from attack from all the modern promoters we throw at them.

For the cells to function effectively, we need our first line of defence – a healthy cell membrane – to be working optimally to: (1) act as an effective protective coating to the cell, i.e. to be a strong castle wall; (2) be a selective barrier, welcoming and wanting necessary nutrients, chemical messages, electrolytes and water, but preventing the entry of unwanted synthetic chemicals and defective chemical messages.

In the same way, a castle wall needs a viable entry, windows and appropriate means of communication with the outside world. On the fatty membrane of any cell is an entire series of surface proteins called receptors, which allow all of these functions. But everything has its limits and once the receptors have been overloaded or unnatural chemicals have attacked the receptors, things start to go wrong.

Antioxidants – are they the real deal?

It is difficult to pick up a magazine, listen to talkback radio, watch a medical-based TV show or even walk down the aisle of a supermarket without seeing some reference to antioxidants.

Antioxidants have been promoted as anything from a useful preventative to a miracle cure for anything from Alzheimer's disease to haemorrhoids. The basic premise of the entire antioxidant argument is that they mop up free radicals – chemicals that have been linked to diseases such as heart and liver disease and cancer. The key to this argument comes from the excessive use of oxygen. If you overload the cell membrane (receptor sites) – the entry point for nutrients and chemical messages into the cell – with either excessive nutrients, synthetic chemicals (which the body was not designed for), radiation or excessive life stresses, as well as creating disordered thoughts and feelings, the chemical reactions created deplete the body of energy. Let's go back to that vital chemical, ATP.

As ATP is vital for the normal function of the cell, once these receptors are overwhelmed by abnormal environmental stressors, the cell then has to increase its normal ATP production to cope with this extra demand on its services.

A direct consequence of this is the excessive use of glucose and oxygen to form ATP, along with a more rapid decay of all the cell's metabolic processes.

Thus, the formation of free radicals. Any time oxygen reacts with nutrients to form ATP, a free radical is formed for every oxygen molecule used. The body has an efficient antioxidant system that mops up these free radicals and returns the radicals back into normal metabolic chemicals that are vital to the normal function of the body.

So, here are the questions that have formed a multi-million-dollar industry known as nutraceuticals, supplements, vitamins, or whatever term you'd like to choose. Do vitamins actually assist the body in neutralising free radicals and are free radicals actually a problem in the first place?

The free radical–antioxidant hypothesis has been around for decades, and I have some good news and some bad news. Let's do the bad news first – I always prefer to finish on a high. The bad news is that free radicals may not have been the actual problem in the first place, but rather a consequence of the problem. Over the past decade, a number of researchers have demonstrated that, rather than being the problem, free radicals are purely the consequence of the initial insult to the body and cells by one of the five factors I've mentioned (i.e. abnormal environmental stimuli such as excessive nutrients, synthetic chemicals, radiation or excessive life stressors, which include disordered thinking and emotions).

Professor Tony Linnane, who pioneered the work with coenzyme Q10, has also been a pioneer in this thinking against the free radical hypothesis. He has shown very elegant work that suggests that, rather than being the initial problem, free radicals are an intricate part of the normal functioning of the cell.

Forget about the Mickey Mouse science, but what Professor Linnane's work has shown is that rather than the free radicals running amok causing all manner of havoc to cellular structures, the free radicals are an integral part of the normal cell messages and are in fact very tightly controlled to ensure that the acid-based balances are within a very narrow range for normal cellular metabolism.

So, rather than use the term 'free radicals' and 'antioxidants', we're probably better off using the term 'signalling'. So, let me introduce a new (but very simple) term – good or bad signals.

Here's a simple scenario to explain my argument. Joe Lipidio books his favourite table at the local Italian restaurant. He is a big boy and enjoys a rather large bowl of pasta. He also has an ample amount of garlic bread, washed down with close to a full flask of the house Lambrusco.

His liver cells are not happy. For the next few hours they're bombarded with excessive nutrients. His receptors for these nutrients on the cell surface become clogged; like four lanes of peak hour traffic merging into two. The receptors are working overtime and begin to make mistakes. Wrong messages or signals are sent to the various parts of the cell, the mechanisms become stressed and the mitochondria (the energy producing part of the cell) is instructed to produce more ATP (energy) to deal with all this overload.

It is somewhat like that age-old TV series *Star Trek*, when Captain Kirk kept asking Scottie to give him more power. The overload also generates more free radicals as a consequence of the initial insult, but if you subscribe to the work of Professor Linnane the free radicals are probably not the issue.

So, the free radical hypothesis is possibly wrong. That is the bad news. Many of us, including me, may have been living under this scientific delusion for a number of years. What's the good news? The good news is that, regardless of the mechanism, the end result is probably not much different. All the usual suspects are still causing major issues in the body. Your metabolic systems are still being over-loaded, damaged and wear out earlier than expected, regardless of the mechanism.

A good example here is diabetes or its forerunner, the metabolic syndrome, and its genetic association, insulin resistance. In all three, the entry of nutrients into the cell is impaired. Insulin's job is to open up the receptors for nutrients on the cell's surface, thus allowing the smooth entry of nutrients across the fatty cell membrane.

In insulin resistance, the door is jammed and the nutrients find it much harder to enter the cell. The body's response to insulin resistance is to make more insulin to force the door open.

Eventually the pancreas (where insulin is produced) says, 'Forget it, fellas, I've had enough,' and starts to struggle to produce adequate amounts of insulin. Levels of fat, sugar and protein start to rise in the blood stream, producing sticky complexes (almost like a toffee apple) called advanced glycosylated end products, or GEPs for short. These sticky, gluggy products produce all types of havoc to cellular metabolism and, not content with screwing around with the cells, also get stuck outside the cells in the walls of blood vessels, leading to atherosclerosis, which, as I detailed earlier in the book, is the major factor causing heart attack, strokes etc.

But let's not stop there: these GEPs also clog up the smaller blood vessels at the nutrient delivery to the organs and thus lead to diabetic, eye and kidney disease, along with a very uncomfortable condition termed peripheral neuropathy.

It all comes back to the major theme of this book. If you use the body for what it was actually designed to do, your body's cells are allowed to function normally.

Throw excessive nutrients, synthetic chemicals or any other form of abuse you can think of at your poor unsuspecting cells and I think you can see what happens.

This now leaves us with another major issue. What about all this antioxidant talk? Antioxidants are supposed to be the white knights that ride in on their chargers saving the day by neutralising the free radicals. However, it has been suggested that free radicals do not need to be neutralised in the first place.

But, stay calm the beating heart of all you vitamin manufacturers, health-food-store owners or leaders of the multi-level marketing companies. Are you peddling snake oil or do these supplements have some function? All will be revealed in the 'To supplement or not to supplement' chapter. I will reveal the good news there.

So, for your cells to be functioning normally, they shouldn't be overloaded with all of the above: you need a healthy, well functioning membrane, high quality macro- and micronutrients delivered across this healthy membrane, along with adequate ongoing amounts of energy.

Now that you understand energy, though, it doesn't actually give you any. In fact, lack of energy, fatigue, tiredness – whatever you'd like to call it – is a problem that affects many people. There are many causes and reasons, which I'll detail in the next chapter.

CHAPTER 5

Fatigue

I've never actually met anyone who has boundless energy and never gets tired. It is the human condition to be tired at various times and for various reasons throughout your life. The feeling of fatigue is your body's way of telling you you either need rest or sleep.

But some people are unusually tired, affecting the quality of their lives. These people need more than a pep pill or a tonic – they need a diagnosis.

The diagnosis of chronic fatigue syndrome is a diagnosis of exclusion. There is no test to confirm this condition and a reasonable definition of this condition is fatigue being present for more than three months with no obvious cause. I'll discuss this condition more fully at the end of the chapter.

There are five other categories of fatigue that need discussion:

1. Stress;
2. Endogenous or chemical depression;
3. Sleep apnoea;
4. The 'pauses';
5. Specific medical disorder.

Stress – moving back to the 24-hour energy allocation I discussed in the last chapter, if you overspend or undercut your allowance in any of these areas, your ATP stores become depleted and you feel tired. So, work 12 hours a day instead of your allocated eight, and you'll feel tired. Run a marathon, and no matter how fit you are, you'll be tired and it will take at least a few days for you to recover. Spend your relaxation time trying to repair broken relationships with those you love, dealing with rebellious teenagers or arguing with disruptive relatives and see where your energy goes.

How many parents with newborns whose sleep is disrupted feel constant high-level energy? How many people who play too hard (with and without added pharmacology, be it legal or illegal) feel good levels of energy, especially when they've come down from this pharmacology?

You're busy at work and you get to bed late and wake up early in the morning to start the cycle all over again. Soon you'll experience burnout. Any of the above and many more life situations contribute to that feeling of fatigue.

These are the first issues I ask about when any of my patients complain of fatigue.

Endogenous depression – this is one of the most common and poorly understood conditions in medicine, both by the public and even some members of the medical profession.

Firstly, it is vitally important to distinguish endogenous depression from grief. Grief is often termed reactive depression by the medical profession. I believe this is a misleading term as it tends to place grief as a medical illness, i.e. depression. If a loved one dies and you feel depressed, in other words you have acutely lost interest in life and feel a sense of helplessness and hopelessness, you are experiencing all the symptoms of grief. It is not depression in the true sense of the word – it is normal to experience these symptoms during such a time of profound loss.

If you didn't feel like this when someone you loved died, I'd say you had something seriously wrong with you, or that there was something seriously wrong with the relationship in the first place. So, when you lose someone or something close to you, whether it be your spouse, a close relative, a friend, a job or even a beloved pet, it is normal to feel grief.

It's good to have the loving support of those around you and you may even need short-term sedatives to help you sleep or calm your anxious feelings, but all manner of cognitive behavioural therapy or antidepressants will not be that helpful in the course of normal grief.

Now, let's bring in the medical illness of endogenous depression. Endogenous depression is an extremely common biochemical disorder of the brain. Twenty per cent of the population will experience endo-genous depression for at least a month during their lifetime. It can manifest itself as everything from a mild disorder to severe, refractory endogenous depression.

The latest theory as to the cause of endogenous depression is a reduction in the brain neuro-transmitter serotonin. Those of us who don't suffer endogenous depression have fluctuating levels of serotonin within the normal range. It is these levels that particularly explain why some days you feel happy and at one with life, but other days you just don't feel like getting out of bed in the morning.

When your serotonin levels drop well below the normal range, endogenous depression starts. The one problem with this theory is that we don't have blood tests to confirm brain serotonin levels. These chemicals work in an instant at the nerve connections known as synapses and we do know that antidepressants increase the amount of serotonin available within the important areas of the brain that determine mood.

The symptoms of endogenous depression are as follows:

1. Fatigue – which is why I've included endogenous depression in this chapter;
2. Early morning wakening. Typically someone with endogenous depression wakes at 2 to 3 am and finds it hard to get back to sleep;
3. Loss of interest in normal activities. This may include work, family activities, libido, sports, hobbies etc;
4. Sense of hopelessness and, in its extreme, suicidal thoughts, attempted suicide and, worst case scenario, successful suicide;
5. Unexplained physical symptoms.

Jean's story

Jean was 77 years old. She was referred to me to investigate her nausea. After extensive investigation of her gastrointestinal tract, her liver and gall bladder, or searching for certain medical conditions through blood tests, I could find nothing wrong.

Jean did have some subtle symptoms of depression, but the nausea was her main debilitating complaint. I commenced her on antidepressants, and within a few weeks her nausea was relieved and she had her old life back again.

We often associate endogenous depression with significant life crises. As mentioned before, many people call their grief 'depression', but this is not really accurate. In fact, when a person's life goes bad this is often because they have developed endogenous depression and they have lost their job because of poor performance.

I'm not suggesting that a serious life crisis cannot result in an episode of endogenous depression, but this must be a medical diagnosis by a skilled practitioner, not an opinion by the person or a caring relative. Actually, the most common cause of an episode of endogenous depression is an unrelated medical illness. Over the past few years, a number of studies have confirmed the association between endogenous depression and heart attack. In fact, one begets the other, i.e. true sufferers of endogenous depression have a much higher rate of acute heart attack and, conversely, the rate of endogenous depression following a heart attack is much higher than one would expect for the normal population. After coronary bypass grafting, 40 per cent of patients develop neuro-cognitive symptoms, of which endogenous depression is a major feature.

Colleen was a woman in her 60s. She had a condition known as unstable angina. The sufferer typically experiences chest discomfort during times of stress, either physical, mental or emotional. This discomfort is relieved when the stress stops. Therefore, if the chest discomfort occurs when someone is walking up the hill, it is relieved when the exercise stops. In unstable angina, however, the pain is more severe, occurs more frequently and often takes place without any obvious cause.

This is a sign to the attending doctor that the person should be seeing a cardiologist rather promptly. Unstable angina pectoris is a medical emergency almost always requiring a coronary angiogram – a dye study of the coronary arteries performed in a hospital.

Colleen was referred to me and I organised a coronary angiogram, confirming severe blockages in her arteries and the need for coronary artery bypass grafting.

Six weeks after the operation, Colleen returned for her routine post-operative visit and, soon after arriving in my consulting room, burst into tears. When I asked her what was wrong, she said, 'You might have taken away my chest pain but now I feel my life is worthless.' Colleen had all the symptoms of endogenous depression. I commenced a short course of antidepressants, returning her serotonin rapidly to normal. When she saw me a month later she thanked me for giving her her life back.

Severe pneumonia, a bad dose of influenza or even a severe physical trauma from an accident may bring on an episode of endogenous depression. One of the most pervasive causes of endogenous depression is cancer, often months to years before the diagnosis of cancer has been made.

Pancreatic cancer is commonly associated with endogenous depression, long before the actual diagnosis is made or any symptoms occur. Thus, in some cases endogenous depression may be the presenting sign of an underlying cancer. Other cancers may also cause endogenous depression without any evidence of tumour in the brain. It is felt that this is due to abnormal signals being released from the localised tumour that directly or indirectly impact on brain function.

So, to approach endogenous depression from the five stages model:

1. *Body Health* – as I've mentioned, at the strictly mechanical level, endogenous depression appears to be an aberration of brain serotonin levels, the therapy being treatment to raise these levels. Although we can't yet pinpoint why, it appears that cognitive behaviour therapy and other forms of counselling and psychotherapy are effective in raising serotonin levels.

    Natural therapies such as St John's wort and Sam-e have been shown in trials to have an effect on mild depression. Although effective, old style anti-depression treatments such as tricyclic antidepressants and monoamine oxidase inhibitors do have significant side effects. SSRIs are very effective in treating endogenous depression, but still have side effects which should be monitored very carefully by the treating doctor.

    This is, of course, not meant to be an exhaustive list of the standard therapies available, more an introduction to the topic.

2. *Environmental* – I'd like to introduce three concepts here that, although discussed on the fringe of this subject, receive little attention:

    a. Diet – serotonin is metabolised in the body from the essential amino acid tryptophan ('essential' means that it must be taken in the diet). Over the past 50 years, we've been bombarded with the nonsense that is the low-fat diet.

Low-fat diets are also typically low-protein diets. Amino acids are the individual components of each protein. Once you swallow any food that contains protein, it's broken down by digestive enzymes in the small bowel to their component amino acids, one of which is tryptophan.

The problem is that if you follow the low-fat, low-protein, high-carbohydrate diet, you reduce your steady supply of tryptophan and therefore your happy chemical, serotonin.

b. Light – one aspect of the entire spectrum of endogenous depression is known as seasonal affective disorder. This is a fancy way of saying that endogenous depression occurs more during winter. One reason for this is the reduced sunlight that occurs, affecting our 24-hour cycle, possibly through the metabolism of melatonin, a neuro-transmitter produced in the pineal gland in the brain.

Some argue it is the change from natural light to artificial lighting since our hunter-gatherer days that affects melatonin metabolism and has an indirect effect on serotonin.

c. Flat screens and other forms of electro-magnetic radiation – I'll discuss this more fully in the chapter on environmental health, but suffice to say that I'm not convinced that long-term exposure to all forms of electronic equipment is good for mental or physical health.

3. *Genetic* – there is no doubt that endogenous depression, in all its forms, runs in families. But if a depressed person brings up

a child, how much of that thought pattern and behaviour is inflicted on the child? Therefore, a depressed parent may be creating a depressing environment in which the child grows up.

4. *Emotional* – as I've mentioned, there is a clear difference between situational grief and endogenous depression, but repeated or severe life crises may also deplete your brain chemicals, plunging you into a clinical episode of depression.

5. *Mind Health* – I'll explain more about this in the final chapter.

In summary, endogenous depression is a common and serious cause of fatigue and needs to be considered when this is proffered as a symptom.

Sleep apnoea – all adult males and all post-menopausal females suffer sleep apnoea to some degree. You may be the type of snorer (snoring is one of the typical signs of the disease) who wakes your neighbours or are so loud that someone might think you're doing rude things with a chainsaw, but there is one question that separates the minor irritations from the serious causes: 'Do you feel refreshed when you wake up in the morning?' If the answer is no, sleep apnoea, or a somewhat related sleep disorder such as restless leg syndrome, needs to be considered and treated.

Common symptoms of sleep apnoea also include marked fatigue (that comes on slowly), daytime semblance and a dry sore throat. There are various treatments for sleep apnoea, but the most important considerations are:

1. Drastic lifestyle changes – weight loss, smoking and alcohol reduction are the keys here;
2. Sleep apnoea jaw splint – wearing this dental mouthguard draws the jaw forward and may improve sleep quality;
3. Nasal CPAP – wearing this mask every night, which pumps air at high pressure to maintain an open airway, is currently the most effective treatment for sleep apnoea;
4. Surgery – various oropharyngeal surgeries have been effective in certain cases in alleviating sleep apnoea, but this needs an initial thorough assessment by an ear, nose and throat surgeon;
5. Pacemaker therapy – innovative researchers at the Austin Hospital in Melbourne have developed a pacemaker procedure that involves monitoring wires on the lung and pacing wires to the tongue buried in a subcutaneous tunnel from a pacing box beneath the collar bone. The box is switched on each night, and with each breath in, the tongue is stimulated, preventing it falling forward and obstructing the airway. This ingenious system has been tested in a number of patients with great success.

It's also important to exclude other medical conditions such as an under-active thyroid and diabetes, which can make sleep apnoea worse.

The 'pauses' – After the age of 40, in both females and males, the gonads, i.e. the ovaries in the females and the testicles in the males, start to lose their optimum function.

This failure in women has been long recognised and termed meno-pause. Over the past 10 to 15 years, a similar condition in males, termed male menopause or andropause, has been suggested (and often refuted by many people in orthodox medicine).

Key features common to both sexes are increasing fatigue, irritability, hot flushes and varying degrees of sexual dysfunction, from vaginal dryness and lack of libido to erectile dysfunction in males. I have a number of patients who say that without their hormone replacement therapy (the mainstay of treatment in men and women), their lives would be worthless. Suffice to say, this period in both women's and men's lives can be marked by significant fatigue and needs to be managed.

Specific medical disorders – before any of the above are accepted as the cause for your fatigue, it's vital that you check whether you have a specific medical disorder. A thorough assessment from a careful physician will be able to determine this.

The most important aspect here is a careful history. How long has the fatigue been present? Did it come on suddenly or slowly? Does it vary throughout the day? Are you short of breath, or do you suffer chest discomfort, dizziness, change in bowel habit? These are a few of the vital questions necessary to determine an underlying medical condition. Once I've performed a history and physical exam, I'll then move on to basic blood tests and other specific tests based on my assessment and the results.

Fatigue is a common feature of many and varied medical conditions. For example, fatigue is a more common symptom of rheumatoid arthritis than joint pain. Fatigue may also be the presenting feature of a heart attack, often days before chest pain or a catastrophic collapse.

I can't remember seeing too many people who've suffered a heart attack who hadn't also – when I applied one of the best medical tests ever, i.e. the 'retrospect-oscope' – earlier suffered fatigue, prior to the event.

Denise was a woman in her 60s. She'd noticed increasing fatigue and shortness of breath over a few months. Her GP referred her to a cardiologist for stress testing. The only abnormality on the test was a marked and rapid increase in Denise's heart rate early on when exercising, without any other changes to suggest blockages in her arteries. The cardiologist diagnosed an atypical form of angina and commenced beta blockers, which have the effect of slowing the heart rate, allowing it to beat more effectively. Rather than feeling better, though, she felt worse, with more fatigue than before she commenced the drugs. (Incidentally, fatigue is a common side effect of many drugs, including beta blockers, and drug therapy of any sort should be included in the differential diagnosis of fatigue.)

Denise came to me for a second opinion. After performing an initial assessment, I ordered a fatigue screen. This revealed that Denise had a marked iron deficiency – anaemia – explaining her fatigue and shortness of breath. Further tests revealed a severe gastritis (inflammation of the lining of the stomach), which was caused by a common gut infection called helicobacter.

The helicobacter was cured with a combination of antibiotics and anti-ulcer treatment. Her blood was restored with oral iron and in a few months her symptoms had disappeared.

As with all issues in medicine, the first step is always to make a diagnosis.

Chronic fatigue syndrome

Chronic fatigue syndrome has been called by many names: Royal Free disease, named after the epidemic of fatigue that occurred in the staff of the Royal Free Hospital in London; post-viral syndrome; yuppie flu, and myalgic encephalomyelitis.

I had one patient who told me she suffered CFS and ME. When I asked her the difference she authoritatively informed me that CFS is when you feel tired all the time and ME is when you feel you have a fog in your head.

In medicine, the true lack of knowledge about the cause and treatment of any condition is related to the number of theories and suggested treatments. The more of both, the less is known. From this point on, I'll drop the other names and call it CFS.

Some of the proposed theories for CFS are as follows:

1. *Post-viral immune disorder* – a person is afflicted by a virus, often glandular fever, otherwise known as Epstein-Barr virus, and has an abnormal immune reaction that attacks the body in particular muscles. A recent study of a chronic viral illness known as xenotropic murine virus (XMLV) was found in 87 per cent of patients with chronic fatigue syndrome, but only 7 per cent of healthy donors. There was also a disturbing link between this virus and prostate and breast cancer. Many studies have failed to confirm this XMLV–CFS link.

2. *Environmental toxins* – many people claim varying reactions to modern society, including chemical sensitivities, reaction to moulds or even problems with electro-magnetic radiation.
3. *Brain disorder* – some MRI studies have demonstrated abnormalities in the areas of the brain that receive energy. However, this may be a consequence, rather than the cause of the disease.
4. *Heart disease* – the American cardiologist Dr Paul Cheney is convinced CFS is a primary cardiac disorder. He argues his case elegantly in a comprehensive lecture that can be downloaded from the internet and it is worth some consideration. Of course, as they say, if all you have is a hammer, everything looks like a nail, and so it is not surprising that a cardiologist would offer this theory.

There has been a veritable cocktail of medications, vitamins and other nutraceuticals suggested for the treatment of CFS. I remember, early in my specialist days, a senior professor in immunology treating CFS patients with intravenous gamma globulin. This was a rather dramatic and potentially dangerous treatment with unproven scientific benefit.

However, the next time you feel tired, you are probably just that – tired! We all get tired for a variety of reasons and this only needs to be investigated if it becomes an ongoing problem. As you can see, though, ongoing and recurring fatigue may often be a manifestation of an underlying serious condition.

CHAPTER 6

Aging – can we stop the clock?

At present, the only way to avoid growing old is to die prematurely. Not a great alternative. The problem with growing old, however, is that the end result is still death, with often decades of various bits breaking down, wearing out or turning nasty in some way.

So the only real solution is to deal with the aging process as best you can. A recent survey of people below the age of 30 suggested they would be happy to live to around the age of 70.

Interestingly, when people aged 79 were surveyed, virtually all of them said they'd be happy to live for many more years. Basically, when you hear the wings of the angel of death flapping around your ears, you really would like a bit more time. The key here is to make this quality time.

So we must ask ourselves: is quality aging and longevity purely good luck, or are there factors that we can influence by our behaviour? I often say that it's your genetics that loads the gun, but it's your environment that pulls the trigger.

There's no doubt that some people are born with lousy genetics and unless their condition is detected early and specifically treated, they'll meet an early demise. Very occasionally, there are also people who stress themselves to the eyeballs and, no matter what modern rubbish they put into their system – such as all manner of processed packaged food, cigarette smoke, excessive alcohol – they'll still survive to a ripe old age and continue to antagonise whomever they have tried to antagonise throughout their lives.

The reality is, however, that most of us are somewhere in the middle. There will be some contribution to our life from genetics, but an equally important contribution from our environment and the way we've looked after ourselves during our time on this earth.

Recently, I saw a patient who'd started to suffer chest pains in her mid-30s, culminating in her having a stent inserted in one of the main arteries in her heart in her early 40s. She told me that the reason for this was her extremely traumatic life, especially the fact that she came from a very dysfunctional family. On further questioning, however, her father also suffered a heart attack in his 40s and died in his mid-50s.

There are definitely strong genetic factors at play here that have contributed to this lady's premature disease, but I have no doubt that her emotional status had also contributed to her significant problems.

There are, though, pockets of people throughout the world who do experience significant longevity. The longest living races or groups on the planet all practise the same thing – it's called moderation. The Okinawans (who live on the island of Okinawa in Japan) have the highest rate of centenarians, i.e. people who live beyond the age of 100. The typical proportion of people who reach the age of 100 is one in 10,000, but they have around 13 to 16 per 10,000 living to this ripe old age, when I suspect they receive the telegram (if they still exist) from the Emperor. The major principle of their eating practices is known as Hara Hachi Bu. It sounds very exotic, but it actually means eating until you are 80 per cent full.

When I first heard this I said to myself, 'This sounds rather sensible,' but then I thought, 'Wait a minute. How on earth do you actually know when you're 80 per cent full?'

Just imagine the conversation at the home of Mr and Mrs Mitsubishi, long-time residents of Okinawa. 'Did you enjoy dinner, Hobi-sun?' 'Yes, very much, but I'm only 73 per cent full and would really like to make up that last 7 per cent ...'

I'm imagining a little 'full-o-meter' strapped to their wrists that monitors gastric fullness. 'Eighty-three per cent – damn, I'll have to avoid the Hara Hachi police!' I think you get the picture. The bottom line here is: don't eat so much.

In third-world countries, it is not unusual for people to survive only to their 30s or 40s. I think the reason for this is fairly obvious.

A major factor in people living beyond 100 is that they have a supreme repair and maintenance system. I don't know about you but I'm not willing to take the one in 10,000 chance of living that long without having a quality lifestyle, as well as consuming high-quality supplements throughout my life.

So, is there a secret to eternal youth which keeps us living well beyond our expected time on this earth? I'm always bemused by patients who assume that because both parents lived well into their 80s that they'll do the same. Unfortunately, those people lived in a different era and were exposed to an entirely different set of life circumstances, environmental poisons and numerous other factors. Just because both parents were 'long livers' (which, I must say, is a very good starting point) does not absolutely guarantee you will be the same.

For example, if you're a smoker and one of your parents smoked and is still alive in their 80s, please don't assume that the same thing will happen to you – because it probably won't. If you do have longevity in your family, this should be an even greater reason for you to want to maintain the trend.

Also, always be suspicious of the miracle cure! When any person, salesman, friend or even a health practitioner suggests that a particular product will cure anything from dementia to haemorrhoids, be very suspicious. Consider the following commonly used arguments.

A particular liver tonic is excellent to cure hangovers. The tonic is taken from a pig liver extract, complete with wonderful testimonials from many regular drinkers. The argument used here is that pigs never complain of a hangover and this liver extract will tune up your liver and make you much less susceptible to the damaging effects of alcohol.

Although what I'm suggesting here is obvious rubbish, many scientific arguments used by quasi-health professionals don't get much better than this either.

So 'natural cures' are very appealing. The placebo response is a well described medical phenomenon. If you give a sugar pill to a person and tell them it has active ingredients in it, the sugar pill has a 40 per cent chance of having an effect.

Interestingly, those people who have great faith in their doctors will respond better to treatment than those who don't. This is not because people are gullible but because of the well-described placebo response.

Another so-called miracle is the story about small pockets of the world where people live to the age of 130 to 140, and despite achieving this extraordinary longevity are still riding horseback, exercising regularly and, while these people have never heard of Viagra, they're still able to make love without any problems.

'I'll be in that,' you might be thinking. Is there any proof behind this story? Do these people really have the secret to eternal youth? There are indeed small pockets of the world – such as the Hunza Valley in Pakistan and areas of Georgia, near Russia – where people maintain they have achieved extraordinary longevity.

So what is their secret? It's very straightforward – birthday parties! Albert Einstein once said: 'Sit with a pretty woman for an hour and it seems like a minute, sit on a hot stove for a second and it seems like an hour – that is relativity!'

Time is a very relative commodity and, in fact, living in areas such as the Hunza Valley or Georgia is really quite boring. From a social viewpoint there is nothing much to do.

So these people, who maintain they are 110 when they look around 50, fill their time in by having birthday parties. Yes, you heard me – the secret to eternal youth is to have more birthday parties than just the one per year. So someone who looks like they're about 50 but maintains they're 110 is, in fact, closer to 50 years old.

The second-oldest recorded living person (with a birth certificate) was Jeanne Louise Calment, who died in Paris around 10 years ago, aged 122. At the age of 121, she recorded a rap dancing song. This next detail is like putting a knife in a cardiologist's chest and twisting it, but when she was 120 she gave up smoking because she said it was becoming too much of a habit.

In 1900, the average life expectancy was around 50 years. In reality, much of this was due to a very high infant mortality rate, but most people who died prematurely died of some type of infectious disease.

In 2010, the average life expectancy had skyrocketed to the late 70s for males and early 80s for females. This is, of course, quite variable. If you examine the longevity rates in third-world countries, these are much lower because of people's susceptibility to infections. Why are they so vulnerable? Because they're malnourished.

You need a certain amount of fat to maintain the integrity of the covering of your cells (known as membranes, as I've mentioned).

These cells are 75 per cent fat and that's why the 30-year mantra of conservative nutritionists and cardiologists about a low-fat diet is absolutely wrong. Low-fat foods and low-fat eating deplete the membranes of fat and make you susceptible to all manner of infections and possibly even cancers. Good-quality fats from natural sources are very important to maintain this membrane integrity and protect you from infectious and inflammatory disease.

However, it's extremely important to achieve a balance with the food you eat. In my book *The Cell Factor*, I explained the problem with consuming modern, processed, packaged food and the synthetic fats that destroy our cell membranes, with help from processed carbohydrates.

You can learn so much from wise, older people. One consultation I'll never forget was a few years back when this wonderful man by the name of Luigi strode into my clinic and sat down. I looked at him, glanced at his birthdate and said, 'Luigi, there must be some mistake – it says here that you're 91 years old.'

Luigi looked at me and said, 'Yes, Doctor, that's correct – I am 91 years old.' I asked him his secret and he replied, 'Doctor, you have got to have a passion.' He then went on to tell me that he had won 2000 awards for growing orchids and 13 world gold medals. Orchids were his passion and had been for most of his life. I examined Luigi and he checked out fine and I reassured him that his heart was as strong as an ox.

Twelve months later he returned for another check-up. I remarked to him, 'Luigi, you don't know how many people I've told about your 2000 awards and your 13 world gold medals.' He looked at me, horrified, and said, 'Doctor, 14!'

Having a passion and setting yourself aside from the crowd is a vital part of longevity. Become what the American psychologist Abraham Maslow described as a no-limit person. Do something because it switches you on and not because it is going to impress anyone else. The huge joy of achieving your goal should become an end in itself.

The compliant members of the tribe are usually subscribers to mediocrity. They tend to retire at the prescribed time, develop their illnesses in their 60s and 70s and move on to the next world right on cue.

Going back to the various populations who exhibit longevity; firstly, the Okinawans not only eat small portions of food, they also keep lifelong friends and find purpose in their life. The Sardinians drink red wine in moderation, share the work burden with their spouse and eat Pecorino cheese and other foods full of omega three fatty acids. The Adventists eat nuts and beans, observe the Sabbath and have faith, and all three groups don't smoke, put family first, are active every day, keep socially engaged and eat plenty of fruits, vegetables and whole grains.

So the next question: why do we age? There are a number of theories to explain aging. Here are just a few:

1. *A free radical–antioxidant imbalance* – a number of researchers, supplement companies and multi-level marketing leaders have built their careers on this hypothesis. Many people all over the world swallow buckets of antioxidants every day in the hope this will afford them tremendous longevity, but I have already argued that the free radical–antioxidant hypothesis may not be scientifically valid. This doesn't mean that so-called antioxidants may not have beneficial effects in other areas.

2. Other researchers have argued that once your hormones start to drift off into the never-never, i.e. menopause and andropause, these abnormal states start to wreak havoc within your metabolic system and your cells start to age at a much faster rate.

3. *Telomeres* – I have previously described these little caps of DNA that keep your DNA packed into a tight ball, so it can snugly fit inside your nucleus and stop the ends from fraying. With each cell division, these telomeres shorten and over time your DNA feels the effects and slowly breaks down, mutates and wears out. This microcellular process also manifests itself as the macroscopic process of aging. You look and feel older, just as your DNA looks and feels older and behaves older, for that matter. All toxins – the usual suspects I keep stressing (stress, of course, being one of them, in all its forms) – speed up the aging

process by affecting your cellular mechanisms, almost certainly through the excessive utilisation of energy, taking the energy away from normal metabolism, where it should be working in the first place as the cells' fuel.

4. *Metabolic syndrome* – a particular form of accelerated aging is the metabolic syndrome I've previously mentioned. This state is characterised by excessive levels of insulin and cortisol, both hormones driving metabolism.

So can aging be stopped, reversed or prevented? I believe the straightforward answer here must be no, but it doesn't mean it can't be affected.

The only specifically proven principle of anti-aging to date has been calorie restriction. It has been proven on multiple occasions in laboratory animals and insects that restricting calories improves longevity, along with signs of aging.

A small, hardy group of human beings – calling themselves the calorie restrictors – has adopted this activity. A major proponent of this rather restrictive lifestyle was Professor Roy Walford. The professor wrote a number of books, the most notable being *The 120 Year Diet*. Strangely, he was taken off the planet at the age of 79, hardly excessive longevity – in fact, it's the average life expectancy of most males in modern society. In the meantime, he had to put up with restricting his calories.

Calorie restrictors look anorectic – because they are – and constantly feel tired and cold. They are also (you'll be shocked when you hear this one) always hungry. Someone should buy them a whip so they can flog themselves as well.

My strong suggestion to you is not rocket science, but it is the theme of any sensible expert in the area of health advice – moderation in all things. No-one should overeat, but I'm certainly not advocating undereating either.

So, what else is on the anti-aging horizon? A big player over the past decade has been *Resveratrol*, a substance that comes from the skin of red grapes. The main action of Resveratrol is that it switches on a group of longevity genes known as sirtuins.

Because it occurs in red grapes, there is Resveratrol in red wine. However, work from Harvard has suggested that the amount of Resveratrol in red wine isn't enough to have a major effect on switching on your sirtuin metabolism.

You can also take Resveratrol as a supplement. Most supplements contain around 300 milligrams, but most scientific studies have used the equivalent of 1000 milligrams daily to demonstrate the switching on of the sirtuin gene. Regardless, the Resveratrol work looks extremely promising and appears to have the same effect as calorie restriction without the misery of being constantly tired, cold and looking like a contestant from *Survivor*.

Another recent advance in the field of anti-aging comes from the unlikely place of Easter Island. This island in the Pacific Ocean is more famous for its enormous stone statues than for its soil. However, living in the soil there is a microbe called *Streptomyces hygroscopicus*, which secretes a very powerful anti-inflammatory immune suppressant known as *Rapamycin*.

Rapamycin has been used over the past decade to coat coronary stents to prevent a strong reaction against them by the arteries called restenosis. It has also been used as an anti-rejection drug for people undergoing kidney transplants.

But, surprisingly, it has also recently been shown to prolong the life of laboratory rodents by up to 30 per cent by switching on an enzyme system known as m-TOR. Although its strong effect on the immune system makes it difficult to use in humans for the purpose of slowing down the aging process, certain tweaks of the molecule may in the future switch on the anti-aging properties without knocking the immune system for a six.

Astragalus is a Chinese herb used for a number of years for a variety of reasons, including anti-aging. A company known as TA Sciences has developed a compound TA-65, which comes from the Astragalus, and which is claimed to induce and maintain telomere length. You will remember that the shorter your telomeres, the shorter your lifespan. It hasn't been studied in long-term human trials to determine its longevity benefit and it is very expensive. However, if it's able to lengthen telomeres then it may be an extraordinary advance in the field of anti-aging medicine.

FIVE POINT CELLULAR ATTACK

1. Accumulation of junk – every time a cell divides, every time a cell does its job, which is either to produce proteins, metabolise nutrients, move (if you are a muscle) or conduct impulses if you are a nerve, the mechanisms involved produce a variety of waste products that need to be removed or reincorporated in the cellular processes.

There are three basic waste products that in turn affect and damage the normal cellular functions.

a. AGEs, Advanced Glycation End Products – excess glucose fat and protein which is not used by the cell becomes stuck or cross-linked together and then stuck outside the cell.

b. Amyloid – although this is a different type of protein which is typically associated with Alzheimer's disease, it basically has the same effect. Amyloid proteins also get stuck around and outside the cells and the connective tissues, affecting the function of cells, the tissues and then the organs.

Within the cell a similar process occurs, where intra-cellular junk known as lipofuscin does the same thing. It goes back to another theme of this book: as is the micro-cosm, so is the macrocosm.

The internal and external accumulation of this junk is exactly the same as you not performing regular home maintenance. If you don't clean your house regularly, keep it tidy and take out the garbage, see how long your house remains functional. If you don't maintain your yard and garden, soon the natural elements of your environment will cause the usual mischief and not only will your home look abandoned, you won't be able to move in and out of your property because of the long grass, fallen branches etc. I think you get the picture and it's not difficult to relate this back to exactly what happens in the cell.

So, of course, we have mechanisms in place to clear this junk but with time and the numerous creative forms of self-abuse humans have discovered along the way, the junk doesn't clear as well as it did, thus aging.

Every aspect of cellular metabolism, including our immune or surveillance/defence system, wears as we age, which is really the mainstay of the system that keeps the junk out of the cells. Within each cell we also have the garbage disposal/recycling centres known as the lysosomes, and like everything else in the body (just for the same reasons), they lose their function and efficiency with time.

All of the above, along with the regular cell divisions that must occur to maintain life, the DNA in your nucleus and mitochondria also become defective as we age.

The field of anti-aging medicine is developing a number of very creative methods to hit the aging process from different angles. Apart from the areas already mentioned, there is a big push to develop a variety of drugs and related substances that break down and clear the cellular junk more effectively.

CHAPTER 7

Controversies and medical myths

Apart from death, the only other certainty in life is that nothing is certain. Nowhere is this more true than in the world of medicine. How often over the past 20 to 30 years have well-respected experts proclaimed, with great certainty, that the cause of this disease is X and the management of this problem is Y, only to be refuted by newer scientific evidence a few years later.

Science and medicine are only as good as their testing equipment, and thankfully, this improves over time. Embarrassingly, though, we experts are also often proved wrong over time.

That's why I'd like to comment on some current controversies and myths and examine the current orthodox view, and of course give my own angle on this area.

Let me make the vital point that I'm not suggesting I'm right – I'm purely giving my opinion from the perspective of someone who's been in the 'thick of it' for over 30 years. Although there are controversies in every aspect of medicine – and life for that matter – I'll focus on areas that affect our day-to-day health. One of the major areas I'll concentrate on is that of supplementation. Should we be supplementing with additional micronutrients or is a healthy lifestyle enough? Are antioxidants the real deal and are free radicals the real evil we've been led to believe?

There is also still a lot of controversy as to whether people should or should not be screened early for disease, how they should be screened, and what tests they should have. So should you be screened at all? If so, when should you be screened, how often and what should you be screened for?

Earlier, I mentioned the saying, 'If all you have is a hammer, everything looks like a nail.' One of the major hammers we have in medicine is a script pad, and a significant number of doctors believe that drugs are the answer to the vast majority of health complaints.

Although pharmaceutical drugs have been powerful in affecting the course of many illnesses, they often have serious side effects and are often over-prescribed. Again, I'll detail where I believe this occurs and what I think should be done about it.

One of the most important aspects of life is to ask questions. Don't accept what you're told without an adequate explanation that sounds feasible. There are often a variety of explanations, approaches and solutions to medical issues.

There is no doubt that, with time, there will be new and better approaches which will replace our current therapy, but suffice to say, many of these suggested treatments are only one aspect towards becoming healthy.

The famous magician David Copperfield has spent his life using illusion to stun his audiences. Some have suggested he used some form of illusion to catch Claudia Schiffer! I'm not sure this relationship is still in existence, but regardless. Although we know it's not real, we still say, 'That's magic.' I'm often bemused when I'm away from my office or an office setting and I hear the call, 'Is there a doctor in the house?' Typically, the doctor rushes to the person in a social setting, a restaurant, a sporting event or at times on the street or a car accident.

The doctor probably isn't carrying his 'tools of the trade' and at best can offer limited first aid; at times, no better than anyone else with adequate training in the ABC of emergencies. I'm often reminded of the television show *Thank God You're Here!* – it's something that's been said to me on the occasions that I've been called to assist in these 'off-site' medical dilemmas.

Strangely, on a few occasions, my extra medical expertise and training has provided that extra bit of magic that would have been otherwise lacking.

'The ball's in your court'

When I was a younger physician, I'd always play squash on a Friday afternoon with a medical colleague. We both avoided the typical medical stereotype of the Wednesday afternoon golf game.

One Friday I walked on to the courts expecting my usual competitive hit-out, when the two gentlemen who always played the hour before us were outside the court. One was standing over the other, who was flat on his back looking very distressed.

He was conscious, sweating (not an unusual finding near a squash court) and totally alert. When I asked him what was the problem, he said his heart was racing. He had no pain, was slightly short of breath, was flat on his back and was not dizzy.

I timed his pulse at 220 beats per minute, typical of what we term supraventricular tachycardia. I immediately commenced a technique known as left carotid sinus massage over his left carotid artery. I also advised him to perform a Valsalva manoeuvre (placing his fingers over his nose and straining hard against his fingers as if he was popping his ears). Within seconds, he'd magically returned to a normal rhythm, felt better, and thereafter he believed I was some type of wizard with mystical hands.

Without wanting to bamboozle you with science, I basically used my knowledge of anatomy and medical training to return this man rapidly back to normal heart rhythm.

These gratifying experiences are quite rare and, more typically, you see a doctor leaning over a collapsed patient pretending to do something meaningful and to ensure that the person in question doesn't require CPR, isn't actively bleeding or doesn't have some other issue that requires basic first aid.

The reason for this longwinded diatribe is that much of what happens in medicine is illusion and often purely a way of managing symptoms. A vast percentage of the medical investigations we perform turn out to be normal. Why are they done? Partly for the very important reason of reassurance for patients and partly for the more defensive reason of covering your butt. A number of lawyers have built their careers on medical errors, omissions and misconceptions. But can I make the very important point that doctors should do a test because they need to, not because they can.

Patients often measure the thoroughness of a doctor by the number of tests that are ordered. The best test you can perform on a patient is to take a thorough and complete medical history and perform a painstaking physical examination. Ninety per cent of medical assessments should be around these two simple principles and any tests should, typically, be used to confirm the doctor's suspicions.

Donald's story

Donald was an overweight 70-year-old insurance salesman who came to see me for an assessment. Prior to his visit, Donald had had a calcium score of his coronary arteries and his score was 800. This placed him in the highest risk group even for a man of his age. I performed a test known as a stress echocardiogram to determine whether he had any blockages in his arteries. The high calcium score tells you that you have a substantial amount of fat in the walls of your arteries but doesn't tell you whether any of this fat has ruptured through to cause a blockage. Donald's stress echo showed some minor slowing in the front wall of his heart consistent with a modest blockage in what is known as the left anterior descending artery.

For a man with no symptoms, who was clearly overweight, with high blood pressure and high cholesterol, a lifestyle change, blood pressure treatment and management of his cholesterol was all that was necessary at that stage.

I sent a report back to his general practitioner, who I didn't know. Donald had been sent to me in the first place through a surgical colleague.

Donald's GP said to him, 'I don't know this Walker bloke. Why don't you see my cardiologist?'

The other cardiologist then performed a stress test (without the echocardiogram). The cardiologist could have easily rung my rooms and I would have been delighted to send him all of the information but he chose not to do so. A stress test is much less accurate than a stress echo and his stress test showed some changes which were also present on the one that I performed, which was no great surprise.

Because of these changes, the cardiologist then proceeded to perform an intravenous CT coronary angiogram (which I totally object to in this setting as it is far too much radiation and does not give any extra information over the stress echo and the calcium score). The intravenous CT angiogram suggested that he had a 70 per cent block in the main artery in his heart and he was then referred for a nuclear scan of his heart (which gives the same information as the stress echo).

The nuclear scan suggested very much the same as my stress echo that he had some slowing down in the front wall of his heart consistent with a modest blockage.

Because of all of this information, his cardiologist decided to perform a coronary angiogram which showed he had a 50 per cent block in the mid-section of the front artery of his heart, known as the left anterior descending. All of this information was highly consistent with what I found initially on my stress echocardiogram.

When I saw Donald, I told him that he should lose weight, and start taking cholesterol lowering pills, blood pressure pills and low dose aspirin. After this thorough evaluation by the other cardiologist, Donald was given the advice that he should lose weight, and start taking cholesterol lowering pills, blood pressure pills and take low dose aspirin.

Strangely, despite all of this, Donald rang my office and abused my secretary, stating that I didn't do enough investigations on him.

I then wrote Donald a letter explaining to him that with the other cardiologist he had had an extra $10,000 to $15,000 worth of investigations, around a thousand chest x-rays of irradiation, and in the end was given exactly the same advice as I gave him.

Basically, if you do coronary angiograms on most fat 70 year olds with high cholesterols and high blood pressure you'll find some minor blockages in the arteries which do not require surgery but certainly require a change in lifestyle and drug treatment.

So, if the doctor has spent time carefully evaluating your situation, don't be disappointed if you leave the surgery without a form for a blood test, x-ray or prescription. You're probably much better off.

The antibiotics scenario is a typical example. It is winter, your nose starts to run, your throat is sore and you feel unwell. You put up with this for a day or so, but, fed up, you book an appointment with your doctor for proper treatment. The problem is, there is no proper treatment. You probably have the common cold, caused by a virus, and there is no specific antiviral treatment for a cold.

In this setting, antibiotics are actually the worst treatment possible. The argument used to be that your doctor is trying to prevent a secondary infection but, in fact, what the antibiotic does is kill the healthy bacteria living in your body, giving you less chance to fight the cold properly.

There have been no effective 'cold-killing' remedies and if your doctor prescribes antibiotics for an uncomplicated common cold, you should find another doctor. Numerous complementary therapies have been tried in this circumstance with variable results. I must confess that when I feel a cold coming on, I fill up with large doses of vitamin C, garlic, Echinacea and zinc. In my case, it appears to minimise the severity and length of the virus, but this may be pure placebo and certainly doesn't work for everyone.

The reality is that we hardly ever cure anything in medicine. We hear of occasional cures for cancer and antibiotics do have the strong potential in most cases to cure a variety of bacterial infections. However, cardiovascular disease, for instance, is hardly ever cured.

If, for example, you suffer a heart attack, we now have superb state-of-the-art therapies to acutely treat the condition. The quicker you get to a hospital after the onset of symptoms, the quicker a stent can be inserted into your arteries. The quicker the time between symptom onset and stent insertion, the less heart muscle is damaged by the attack.

This is precisely why heart organisations around the world encourage you to ring the emergency line for the ambulance and have you rushed to hospital for immediate assessment. But, after the heroics have been performed with the stented artery and your pain relieved, after a few days or so you're sent back to the situation from whence you came, loaded with a handful of pills to 'thin your blood, lower your cholesterol, keep your heart calm and maintain low blood pressure'. You are certainly very well treated, but definitely not cured.

The underlying process – atherosclerosis – needs to be aggressively treated and in many cases, I believe, may even be reversed. This is a process that very much involves the five stages of health.

Any area of specialty – be it medicine, science, law, technology, or basically any discipline – uses flowery, esoteric language to create magic.

This subconsciously conveys to the consumer of that discipline certain powers that the experts really don't possess.

To give a couple of simple examples from medicine: you visit your doctor and have your blood pressure checked. It is high on a few occasions and the doctor suggests treatment. Any inquisitive patient may ask the following reasonable question: 'Why do I have blood pressure, Doctor?'

'You have idiopathic hypertension!' replies the doctor.

'Oh … thank you,' replies the patient, satisfied with the diagnosis. Basically, however, idiopathic means we don't have a clue what causes it and hypertension is not heightened stress, but purely high blood pressure. The reality is that in 90 per cent of cases of hypertension, there is no known cause apart from the combination of multiple common genetic factors, combined with the abnormal environment of our modern society.

When I was training as a specialist, I spent six months working for a world-famous neurologist before focusing on my chosen specialty – cardiology. This brilliant man had a velvet soothing voice, an unsurpassed knowledge of neuroanatomy and was a superb diagnostician. But there was a problem. Over 30 years ago, many neurological conditions had no specific treatment, often leaving the sufferer with a progressive, debilitating, long-term condition.

The presence of the professor at the bedside, wielding his tendon hammer and then suggesting some diagnosis, often with a string of ancient neurologists' names strung together, would cast some magic over the patient and their relatives, despite the fact that this performance made absolutely no difference to the person's long-term outcome. That's the magic of medicine!

CHAPTER 8

To supplement or not to supplement

I recently received a phone call from relatives of a man in his 90s who had been admitted to a major teaching hospital in Sydney, almost demanding that I visit this man whom they believed was being mismanaged.

This was despite the fact that I'd never laid eyes on him or his family before and knew nothing of his case. My bemused PA – who, thankfully, shields me from these types of intrusions – related the details of the situation as given to her by one of this elderly man's distraught relatives.

He had a heart condition but the specialists caring for him had stopped all of his supplements. The man's family believed that this intervention by the treating cardiologist had contributed to his deterioration. They'd heard that I believed in using both traditional (or orthodox) medical techniques and Complementary and Alternative Medicine, and they felt that if I intervened and reinstituted his 'natural therapies', all would be restored, his health would magically return and yet another life would be saved!

As well as the fact that I had no visiting rights to this particular hospital and therefore it would be illegal and, of course, very unethical for me to interfere with my colleague's treatment of any patient, I find some people's blind faith in natural medicines and their opposition to scientifically validated orthodox medicine quite bizarre, not to mention the fact that they felt they had the right to ask someone they'd never met to intervene on their behalf.

This chapter is about perspective. While, in many cases, there is certainly a place for supplementation, as I mentioned earlier in the book I don't believe that supplements are miracle cures, wonder drugs that can be used instead of proven, conventional medical therapy. That's why they're called supplements. They are supplements to ongoing lifestyle practices and – where necessary – appropriate medical and surgical intervention.

So, what is the place of all three: lifestyle, supplements and orthodox medical treatments? Firstly, lifestyle is king. Without my five keys to a healthy life, you're really starting well behind the eight ball.

I've previously mentioned the five key lifestyle principles in increasing order of importance: (1) maintain ideal body weight/weight circumference; (2) have no addictions; (3) good quality, natural food and less of it; (4) at least three hours per week of testing exercise; (5) happiness, peace and contentment.

These five magic principles reduce your risk for all diseases by somewhere between 60 to 70 per cent.

You derive around 25 to 30 per cent additional benefit from orthodox medicine and, depending on the mix, around 5 to 10 per cent from supplementation. Therefore, putting supplementation into the equation, it is certainly the least important of all of our interventions.

I've mentioned that I'm always staggered by people who are prepared to bombard their bodies with a multitude of pills or swallow a bucket of vitamins, but continue to smoke or (just as bad) look like something Greenpeace would try to push back out to sea. So please, before you even start on whether you should or shouldn't supplement, get your health in the correct perspective. I see supplements as an effective (albeit relatively weak) health preventative manoeuvre and, just like excellent lifestyle habits, they work over the long term, not just a few years.

So, getting back to the original story, was there any sound medical reason for me to ride in on the white steed to this major hospital and demand that the supervising cardiologist reinstitute this elderly man's supplement therapy? Absolutely none!

Supplements in perspective

It's estimated that well over half the population in the modern world have either sought the help of a complementary therapist or have taken some form of complementary medicine during any one year.

Complementary and Alternative Medicine (CAM) is defined as a group of diverse medical and health-care systems, practices and products that are not generally considered part of conventional or orthodox medicine. Basically, these are all the rest, when you exclude what we see as pharmaceutical therapy, surgical and medical interventions. I'd also like to exclude other conventional therapies such as physiotherapy, speech pathology, dieticians, exercise physiologists and occupational therapy from CAM.

So, CAM includes – and this is not an exhaustive list – the prescription of natural products, mind-body (including energy) medicine, and manipulative and body-based practices.

Many orthodox doctors, however, use some CAM therapies, and many of them use the term 'integrative medicine' to describe their methods. At a recent dinner in Australia for the National Institute of Integrative Medicine, Professor Avni Sali – who is a great friend of mine – introduced me as the guest speaker. He made the comment that I was the only integrative cardiologist practising in Australia. Although I was proud to accept the title, I felt it was rather sad if this was true.

I believe, as practising doctors, we all should be trying to take the best parts of orthodox and complementary medicine to offer our clients the best integrated services.

But this chapter is all about whether there is any validity in supplementation. Firstly, let me mention the concept of deficiencies. Anyone living in a modern, developed society who consumes a reasonable diet, including a modicum of fruit and vegetables, and who doesn't have an underlying disease (like celiac or pernicious anaemia, to give two examples) will not have a deficiency state.

While there are very few cases of micronutrient deficiencies seen in our modern, developed community, the same cannot be said for many inhabitants of Africa, India and other parts of Asia. It also cannot be said for sufferers of anorexia nervosa.

I have many patients say to me, 'But, Doctor, I have a healthy diet with plenty of fruit and vegetables – why do I need a vitamin?'

A legitimate question deserves a legitimate answer. There's no doubt that you receive enough micronutrients, i.e. vitamins, minerals and trace metals, in a typical modern diet. And if you're not swallowing vitamins to make up a deficiency, why bother? I believe the reason we should bother is that there's evidence that they improve metabolic regulation in a number of ways.

For all the reasons I've argued in the preceding chapters, our normal metabolic processes wear out and deteriorate as we age. The consequences to our bodies include:

i. Energy – increasing loss of energy and fatigue;

ii. Metabolic changes – the general effects of metabolic slowing which leads to the increasingly frequent manifestations of the metabolic syndrome, e.g. a tendency to diabetes, hypertension, increased cholesterol, abdominal obesity and cardiovascular disease;

iii. Specific effects of cardiovascular and respiratory systems – as we age, the protein elastin is replaced by the stiffer protein collagen, stiffening our blood vessels, leading to hypertension and a stiff heart itself. There is also loss of elastic tissue in the lungs leading to much less efficient intake of oxygen and output of carbon dioxide, among other issues;

iv. The hormonal system – directed by the pituitary gland at the base of the brain and involving a series of areas throughout the body including the thyroid, the adrenals, the gonads (ovaries in the female and testes in the male) along with the pancreas are certainly affected by the ravages of recurrent daily and monthly cycles and then also changes from wear and tear over decades.

This has obvious ramifications with menopause and the somewhat disputed male version, andropause. There are a variety of other disease processes that may affect these glands, but suffice to say still related to some aberration in the wear and tear process.

v.   Kidneys – as the major filter of the blood, as you can imagine it doesn't take much for this toxic assault to stuff up the vital kidney filtering mechanism. Toxins and all the aforementioned cellular junk may clog the filter, leading to progressive kidney damage, an increasing problem in our modern world.

vi.   Skin – as we age, the skin becomes thinner, loses its elastic properties and the blood supply becomes very friable, leading to subcutaneous bruising. Many people are appropriately taking some form of aspirin, which makes this skin bruising so much more common. Add to this, exposure to UV rays over the years and the poor old skin certainly becomes just that.

vii.   Connective tissues – the bones, joints and muscles, i.e. our muscular skeletal system, along with the other connective tissues or supporting structures within the body, are particularly susceptible to wear and tear. There are not too many long-term athletes who haven't suffered some sort of musculoskeletal injury. My own knees are wrecks!

viii. Our immune system – it never sleeps. It's like a security guard looking for trouble. As soon as it finds it, it has to rally the troops to action to sort out the problem. If you imagine a system that has to do this day in day out, well beyond its designated use-by date of 30 to 40 years, you are just asking for trouble.

Thus, there is no doubt that good genetics and an excellent lifestyle are the key, but do supplements offer any added benefits? It's also important to ask: could they possibly do any harm?

'High dose vitamin E death warning'

This was a headline on the BBC website in November 2004. That month, Dr Edgar Miller had published an article that brought together a number of studies about vitamin E. The paper was entitled 'Vitamin E – A Cause of Increased All Cause Mortality' (or for want of a better word – death). Although vitamin E has been considered for a number of years to be a powerful antioxidant, this may not be the reason for its benefit and may be the downside to its use. It has been firmly established that vitamin E is an antioxidant, but it has other actions which I believe are its key benefits:

Cell signalling – I have introduced the concept of good and bad signals. When a chemical binds to a receptor on the cell membrane, it can either have a good effect inside the cell, i.e. contribute positively to cell metabolism, or it can have a bad effect (a negative contribution), i.e. a good or a bad signal. Vitamin E appears to bind to receptors on the cell surface that leads to membrane stability and protection and thus has nothing to do with its antioxidant capacity. Some authorities argue that vitamin E has minimal antioxidant activity in the body, despite its obvious action in the laboratory.

Vitamin E also has an effect on the sticky cells which assist in clot formation, known as platelets. Therefore, vitamin E may also act as a blood thinner.

In the form of d-alpha-tocopherol, vitamin E appears to have a variable ability to either block or induce tumour growth depending on the type, i.e. alpha-tocopheryl succinate versus nicotinate or acetate.

Overall, it appears that d-alpha-tocopherol has a direct role as a good signal promoter for gene expression unrelated to its antioxidant effect.

Vitamin C enhances the action of vitamin E. These substances combined may prevent a reduced formation of cancer-inducing nitrosamines which occur with overcooked meats, sausages, bacon and delicatessen meats. Like vitamin E, vitamin C has numerous actions outside of its proposed antioxidant role. There is mounting evidence that it is these other actions that provide the real benefit for supplementing with vitamin C. Vitamin C is an essential coenzyme (there go those good signals again) in the production of collagen. It is also important in the production of one of our most important brain chemicals, dopamine. It is also found in high concentrations in the pituitary and adrenal glands.

Vitamin C also appears to inhibit the spread of bacteria and in some studies there was no difference in the conventional markers of oxidative stress between animals supplemented and not supplemented with vitamin C.

Also, it is important to stress the vital promotion of vitamin E action by vitamin C. Another fascinating action of vitamin C that needs to be investigated is the controversial use of intravenous vitamin C. Large oral doses (up to 10 grams per day) of vitamin C did not increase the plasma ascorbate levels above 0.3 millimoles but when the same result was given intravenously this resulted in levels of 6 millimoles. It appears that vitamin C above levels of 5 millimoles acts as a prodrug promoting the formation of high concentrations of hydrogen peroxide which is lethal to a range of human and rodent cancers.

To summarise, here are the vitamin supplements I'd recommend for the following conditions:

1. Energy – coenzyme Q10, 150 milligrams, two daily; as well as magnesium orotate, 400 milligrams, one to two daily (this supplement is particularly important if you're taking statin drugs to lower cholesterol).

2. Metabolic syndrome – chromium, 400 micrograms, especially if combined with cinnamon in either a capsule, or as a typical preparation purchased from a supermarket; Bergamet, purple carrots (I'll explain more about both of these later in the book).

3. Cardiovascular support – a variety of supplements have been shown to provide benefit: fish oil or flax seed, at least 4 grams daily; as well as hawthorn herbal treatment, 600 to 1200 milligrams daily, and vitamin E 500 international units of d-alpha-tocopherol around the evening meal. Also, vitamin C 500 to 1000 milligrams taken with vitamin E around the evening meal.

In another blow to the supplement sceptics, a recent study from Israel treated 70 patients for six months. This randomised controlled clinical trial used vitamin C, 1 gram daily; vitamin E, 400 international units daily; coenzyme Q10, 120 milligrams daily, and selenium, 200 micrograms per day, compared with a placebo.

Arterial stiffness was measured, along with metabolic profile (cholesterol, blood sugar level etc). There was a significant improvement in the treated group over this short period of time. Parameters of arterial stiffness improved, along with a drop in diabetic levels and an improvement in HDL (good) cholesterol levels.

4. Brain – (Alzheimer's disease prevention: folic acid, 800 micrograms; B6, 20 milligrams; B12, 500 micrograms daily) Brahmi/Ginkgo biloba/phosphatidylserine.

5. Hormones – a variety of natural supplements have been proposed. As this is such an individual area and requires full supervision by an expert, I'd suggest seeking a professional opinion if you're significantly affected by menopause or andropause.

6. Gastrointestinal – numerous herbs and detoxification programs have been proposed to maintain gut health. There is also strong evidence for a variety of probiotics.

7. Kidneys – this is a tricky area and unfortunately a handful of people with serious kidney disease have been given dangerous advice by a small group of CAM therapists. There is, in fact, a rarely used Chinese herb, aristolochic acid, which may induce end stage kidney failure.

    If there is any suggestion of kidney disease, you need expert assessment from your doctor.

8. Skin – a variety of supplements are used very commonly in skin creams and lotions which claim to maintain skin integrity and reduce wrinkles.

    A number of supplements, including olive fruit extract, have been shown to concentrate in the skin. In one study there was a 40 per cent reduction in wrinkles using an olive fruit extract.

9. Connective tissues – regarding the muscles, coenzyme Q10 is a specific muscle supplement and it's my opinion that it should be used in the vast majority of people over the age of 40 to 50, unless there is a specific medical contraindication.

10. The blood and immune system – over the years, many experts have suggested a number of natural immune stimulants. I believe the best evidence is for the combination of spirulina and grape seed extracts.

As you can see, it's my position that you gain extra benefits from taking the correct supplements for your condition. It is, though, vitally important you don't make this decision alone. Develop a relationship with a trusted health practitioner and formulate a program that best suits your needs.

The most important point here is: don't lose perspective. Real estate agents often say, 'Location, location and location.' However, the most important 'L' here is 'lifestyle, lifestyle and lifestyle'.

CHAPTER 9

The five-point way to a healthy lifestyle

As I make very clear throughout this book, lifestyle is king. Without a solid foundation of the following five lifestyle principles, it is difficult to stay healthy, and very uncommon. Although I'm presenting the five stages of health, these are all based on the foundation of the five points to a healthy lifestyle. Without a healthy lifestyle, the addition of the five stages has no foundation.

1. Achieve Ideal Body Weight

   We're all constantly bombarded with advertisements for weight-loss programs, wonder diets that strip fat from you faster than the blink of an eye, or the miracle nutritional supplements that can make your belly disappear quicker than a politician's promises. The reality is, there is no magic. I've written five books on nutrition and I can assure you that the only program that works is very obvious and straightforward. It is what I refer to as the in/out principle. Basically, to lose weight you have to take in fewer calories than you burn off every day for the vast majority of your life.

A diet doesn't work because it is finite. Most diets have an average longevity of a month or so. As soon as you stop, the weight pours back on. The important principle here is the amount and timing of each meal and its relationship to exercise. I was once a very strong supporter of the Mediterranean diet, which works beautifully if you have a Mediterranean lifestyle. The difference between someone with a true Mediterranean lifestyle and someone living in Western society is that with a Mediterranean lifestyle you have a solid breakfast, your largest meal is the lunchtime meal, followed by a small evening meal. After your rather large lunchtime meal you have a sleep for an hour and then burn off any excessive carbs by toiling in the fields all afternoon.

In our society, we have a smallish breakfast and lunch with often high-energy, nutrient-poor snacks in between, and then come home and have a rather large evening meal and afterwards sit in front of the television. The body is not like a car. When you put fuel in a car, it can sit in the petrol tank until you next need to use it. If you put fuel in your own 'car', i.e. your body, if you don't burn it off within a few hours, it is laid down as fat, and that fat becomes increasingly difficult to shift.

Also, the system is not particularly kind. If you have a solid half-hour brisk walk, you burn around 300 calories. If you eat one reasonable size piece of chocolate cake, you put on 300 calories. The average intake of someone living in Western society should be somewhere between 2000 and 2500 calories of food per day. If you venture to one of those very popular commercial takeaway food outlets with the golden arches out the front and consume one Big Mac, one thick shake and one regular serve of French fries, you're taking in 1500 calories in one hit. Therefore, you can see it's quite difficult to maintain the in/out principle and keep your weight down.

Tony's story (written by himself)

This chapter of my life started in early December 2006. I was 58 years old, I weighed 165 kg and I was extremely unfit, becoming increasingly immobile. I was so depressed about my condition and general health that I consulted a surgeon and was booked in to have gastric banding two weeks before Christmas. Luckily, I made an appointment to see Dr Ross a week before my surgery. During a very emotional meeting he convinced me that, due to its proximity to Christmas, I should delay the operation until the New Year and in the meantime lose some weight to make the operation easier and safer.

I took that very valuable advice and found myself losing weight the right way, to the extent that I did not have the operation. I continued to lose weight over the next two years and in December 2008 I found myself at 125 kg and was starting to feel great. People were also starting to notice my new shape and were most complimentary. Although I had every intention of continuing to reduce my size, I started to lose urgency and, slowly but surely, weight started to go back on. By the end of 2009 I weighed 141 kg and I was back on the roller coaster ride which I had been on so many times before.

I am in the life insurance and financial planning industry. During December 2009 and January 2010, a series of industry meetings and subsequent events changed my life and, as it happened, also saved it. I attended a meeting with Asteron at which they launched a web-based, health and wellness program for their clients. I was so impressed that following the meeting I wrote to them with promotional ideas to expand the awareness of their program. I suggested they should encourage Sydney identities to participate in the program to lose weight and improve their fitness. At the same time, those people could support local charities by asking people to donate a specified amount for every kilo lost. Their profiles would attract the media and so gain Asteron the publicity they deserved. To my surprise they liked my idea but wanted to promote the program to the industry with me as the face of the program. The thought initially terrified me – I would then be accountable and failure would not be an option – but as I thought about it, I turned the negatives into a huge positive. I accepted their offer on the condition that I could use the opportunity to raise money for Motor Neurone Disease Australia (MND), a charity which is close to my heart.

I have seen three of my friends die from this insidious disease. One, Philip, was like a brother to me. MND is a progressive degenerative disease which affects muscular functions, causing paralysis of voluntary muscles. There is currently no known cause or cure and most sufferers will take between two and five years to die. The disease started in Phil's legs and over a two-year period worked its way up his body until he could no longer swallow or breathe. It is such a debilitating condition and a terrible way to die.

Once I had committed to Asteron, I decided to have a full medical including a visit to Dr Ross, whom I had not seen for four years. He sent me for a cat scan to measure the calcium build-up in the arteries to the heart. From this reading, you can ascertain how much fat there is in the arteries. I knew when I took the results back to him that I was not in great shape but I don't think he wanted to frighten me in case I died on the spot. It was not until I attended a breakfast seminar held by a life insurance company two weeks later that I realised the full extent of my condition. Their chief medical officer talked about this cat scan, attracting my immediate attention. He said with a reading of zero it is unlikely that one would have a heart attack. However, if the reading were 400, he would not buy a copy of *War and Peace*. At that point I pushed my eggs and bacon aside and felt myself turn ashen white. My reading was 782. It scared the living daylights out of me. Suddenly I faced the fact that I could drop dead at any point. I was destined to have a massive heart attack and my life expectancy could no longer be measured in years. All my plans for a happy retirement and growing old with my grandchildren were shattered. I suddenly had another huge incentive to start the Asteron program and make it work.

Apart from giving me a great deal of moral support, Asteron also asked one of the sponsors of their program, Dr Adam Fraser, to assist me to set up my new eating and exercise routine. Adam runs a business called the Glucose Club, assisting obese people and those with diabetes to lose weight and improve their health. His assistance and ongoing support was wonderful. The program aside, Adam kept me focused. He would call me twice a week just to ask how I was going and I sensed every time that he really cared. I would send him once a week a schedule of everything I ate and what my daily moods and energy levels were. I would also report what my exercise for the week had been. In those initial months Adam truly kept me on the straight and narrow. It is very difficult to let down someone who really cares and is going the extra mile for you.

I started the program late in January 2010. At that time I weighed 141 kg and was very unfit. I had high blood pressure, high cholesterol, chronic sleep apnoea, was bordering on diabetic and at severe risk of heart attack. In fact, I was so conscious of my heart problems that I feared going to sleep at night, afraid I may not wake up. Every twitch of a muscle around my chest or neck worried me. Getting through those first few months was very stressful and an experience I never want to repeat.

True to my plan, although slightly delayed, I went to my industry and asked for sponsorship for MND and support for my weight loss. I am pleased to say that the response I received was overwhelming, far exceeding my expectations. By the time the sponsorship started I was down to 131 kg and going well. The combined sponsorship was $462 for every kilo I lost – this was an immense motivator for me to keep losing weight. Every time I was tempted to eat outside my plan, I thought of MND and how much it might cost them. It gave me an urgency that even my health concerns did not create. Especially towards the end of the year when I was getting closer to my goal weight and feeling wonderful, my drive to earn MND as much as I could kept me focused. At the conclusion of the nine months sponsorship period, MND received approximately $18,000.

I would love to be able to give you my program in detail and lend you my magic wand so everyone could enjoy the success that I have had, but unfortunately there is no easy formula or magic. I simply cut back my intake to 1500 calories a day and exercised every day to make sure I burnt up as many calories as I was physically capable of doing. At the start I would walk for 30 to 40 minutes, avoiding as many hills as I could. By the end of the year I was walking one to two hours a day, looking for hills and increasing my speed. I also incorporated an exercise and stretching program which I did every second day.

My weight loss was not rapid but it was consistent and during the first 47 weeks I lost 43 kg. Over that period I have been able to adopt new eating habits and lifestyle routines which will stay with me and ensure I will never go back to my former weight.

Today I am 98 kg. I still have a few to lose but I am off all medication for blood pressure and cholesterol, my sleep apnoea has all but disappeared, my sugar levels are on the low side of normal and a recent ECG would suggest my heart is not about to stop beating. The daily exercise has improved my fitness considerably and, although I do not see myself running a marathon, I reckon I could easily walk one.

Reflecting back, I ask myself why I endured that weight for so long and I do not have an answer. I was recently, however, reminded of a quote from that great man Mahatma Gandhi who said, 'I am the message. It is not what I say, it is what I do.' I have a gorgeous wife and two wonderful grown up daughters, all of whom have a history of excess weight and I have to ask myself what message I have been giving them over the past 30 years and whether it has influenced their weight problems. I am sure the answer is yes. I just hope that the message I am now portraying influences them and others to follow, because there is no doubt that obesity, like smoking, has a huge impact on health and longevity.

Body mass index

The body mass index is a long-used indicator of ideal weight. It has long been said by the medical and nutritional world that a body mass index between 20 and 25 is the healthy range, 25 and 30 is becoming overweight, greater than 30 is obese, and greater than 40 is morbidly obese. There are many flaws in the system and, as one example, a professional athlete with a large muscle mass will have a body mass index which places him in the overweight-to-obese range without an ounce of body fat.

In fact, if you look at the totality of evidence, people with BMIs in the 22–28 range probably have the best long-term health outlooks. Therefore, carrying a little bit of extra fat around the belly is not too dangerous. Probably the best indication of risk is your waist circumference. A waist circumference for a male greater than 95 cm (37.4 inches) and greater than 80 cm for a female (31.5 inches) is above the acceptable risk and something that should be worked on.

David is a male in his late 50s whom I first met at my Melbourne clinic over 12 months ago. At that stage he was significantly overweight, had a high cholesterol, and because of abnormal parameters on my arterial screening test suggesting he was in trouble, I organised further extensive blood testing and a CT scan of his coronary arteries. At that stage David had no symptoms, apart from feeling somewhat tired.

The CT scan of his coronary arteries showed a calcium score of 350, which placed him at moderate risk for a heart attack. His cholesterol was 6.5, he had an elevated Lipoprotein(a) (as I've mentioned, this is a genetic cholesterol-carrying protein that can often deposit fat in your arteries from a very early age), his highly sensitive C-reactive protein, which is a general test of inflammation, was 6.5 (normal is less than 5; ideal is less than 1.5), and his homocysteine, which is an indirect indication of cell repair, was 33 (normal is less than 10; ideal is less than 7).

I must have flicked some switch in his head, because I reviewed him at a recent follow-up clinic in Melbourne and didn't recognise the man. He had lost 23 kg, his cholesterol – on a combination of weight loss and medications – had dropped from 6.5 to 3.5. His highly sensitive C-reactive protein had dropped from 6.5 to 0.4 and his homocysteine had dropped from 33 down to 7. His arterial stiffness had improved and basically he said he felt better than he had for 10 to 15 years.

David's is an amazing case of cardiac reversal. I am more than happy to take some of the credit for this extraordinary turnaround, but I'd place most of this marvellous result squarely on his shoulders. It's easy enough for any doctor to give advice but the human being has to take that advice onboard and do something about it. We all know that often in life the most difficult aspects also offer the greatest rewards. The quick-fix solution to any problem is usually just a Band-Aid on a festering sore and in David's case he has opted for the long-term fix which will give him a much greater benefit.

I am not suggesting he is now at zero risk for a heart attack, but when I initially saw him I would have estimated his 10-year risk to be in the 60 to 70 per cent range, but now with the combination of lifestyle modification, supplementation and the appropriate use of medications, we've reduced that risk to well below 5 per cent.

There is no magic in the program, David is just following a combination of sensible living and the appropriate use of natural and pharmaceutical preparations. This approach is available to us all and it is entirely up to you whether you wish to follow the program – it's not rocket science!

2. Nutrition

There are five key points that need to be discussed in regard to nutrition:

i.   Low-fat nonsense
ii. Convenience is killing us
iii. Paleolithic principle
iv. Body typing
v.   The 19 out of 21 rule

Low-fat nonsense

In the middle of last century, a researcher known as Professor Ancel Keys released the results of a study known as the Seven Countries Study. This was the start of the low-fat message. The evidence basically came from the Japanese race, who traditionally consume a diet relatively low in fat (despite their fish intake) and have a significant longevity and a very low rate of coronary heart disease. Strangely (for reasons I'll present in a moment), the evidence of the people of Crete was overlooked and not seen to be as important as the Japanese experience. The people of Crete and other Mediterranean areas are on a traditionally high-fat diet – but good quality natural fats that actually protect against heart disease.

Despite this, if you ask any person on the street what the best diet is to avoid heart disease, they'll immediately trot out the low-fat mantra. In fact, being on a low-fat diet, and in particular avoiding meat, eggs and dairy, has absolutely no scientific basis whatsoever. It has, however, very much suited the food industry to promote this message as it can promote and sell processed, packaged muck, masquerading as food, in a box or a container.

In 2001, a study released in the *British Medical Journal* reviewed 27 different trials of modifying fat intake, confirming the fact that there is not one shred of scientific evidence that following a standard low-fat diet will prolong your life by one millisecond.

The real mischief-makers in this regard are the food industry, who are subtly poisoning us with low doses of synthetic fats (mainly trans fats), which are used for the purpose of thickening and hardening food. Basically, if it is in a box or a container in a thickened, hardened state, it has a degree of trans fatty acids (with usually a fair bit of carbohydrates, salt and other chemicals), which cause not so subtle problems for your body. So, ladies and gentlemen, the low-fat diet is not healthy and in most cases should not be considered.

Convenience is killing us

One of the unfortunate characteristics in most of us human beings is the desire for a quick fix. Interestingly, amongst the wealthiest people on the planet are those selling instant gratification. Whether it be software manufacturers, oil barons or, in one particular instance, the owner of a worldwide furniture company, it is this instant gratification, the 'I want it and I want it now' attitude, that has made these people extremely wealthy. Human beings love to purchase, they love to consume, but what most don't like doing is putting in the hard yards.

Interestingly, it is the hard yards that are usually most important. Nothing could be more telling than when it comes to our health. I believe this 'quick fix' issue is one of the major reasons we're seeing our current health dilemmas, and that convenience, or the quick fix, is killing us.

As I've mentioned, the true cause of our problem is convenience foods, which are laden with synthetic fats and processed carbohydrates. Basically one of the healthiest things you can do for your family is to go home with a blow torch and get rid of your pantry. If it is in a box or a container with a use-by date in a thickened, hardened state – and personally I don't care what graffiti is written on the side of the box such as 'low fat' or 'no cholesterol' – there are subtle doses of synthetic fats, probably buckets of processed carbohydrates, not to mention the salt and other chemical additives to either colour or preserve the food.

Bakery foods with pastry are also a good source of poison. It is not the meat in meat pies that is killing you – because as you know there is no meat in meat pies – it is the pastry on the outside. One of the greatest oxymorons on the planet is a 'low-fat' muffin. If you have a piece of steak every day, you take in an extra 5 per cent of saturated fat and this translates to around a 17 per cent increase in your risk for a heart attack. Therefore, you should probably not have a piece of steak every day. If, however, you have a donut, a croissant or a low-fat muffin per day, you're having around a 2 per cent increase in your trans or synthetic fatty acid intake and this translates to up to a 93 per cent increase in your risk for a heart attack.

Speaking of quick-fix foods, you might be aware of Morgan Spurlock's contribution to the nutritional world. A few years ago, he decided to eat at McDonald's three times a day for a month, and made a documentary *Super Size Me*. At the end of the month, Mr Spurlock had gained 13 kg, his cholesterol had risen from 3.5 to 7 mm/L and his blood pressure rose from 110/70 to 160/100. The only thing that didn't rise was something that most of us males like to rise occasionally. Yes, you guessed it, after a month of consuming this rubbish, Mr Spurlock had become impotent.

The obvious retort to this is that no-one eats this food three times a day for a month, and of course they don't. But many people consume the equivalent amount over 10 years and have a guess what happens. They put on 13 kg, their cholesterol doubles and their blood pressure goes through the roof. Meanwhile, something else no longer goes through the roof.

I'm not suggesting you should never have takeaway food, but you should very much minimise your intake of this stuff if you really are serious about being healthy.

Another aspect of quick-fix rubbish is the consumption of soft drinks and fruit juices. In the old days, when I was a boy, the government used to supply school children with milk for morning playtime. They'd leave it in the playground, it would get warm, you would drink it and throw up in the corner! Only joking, of course. Basically, we were being encouraged to consume calcium-based products as part of good health.

These days, though, children will have a soft drink or a fruit juice for morning tea. Most of these standard fruit juices have up to the equivalent of 10 teaspoons of sugar, and a recent study showed that people who consume one standard can of soft drink per day have a 50 per cent increase in their risk for diabetes later in life.

Don't think that the diet drinks are much better. Another recent study showed that people who consume three diet drinks a week have a 19 per cent increase in their risk for diabetes, and those who have three diet drinks per day have an 87 per cent increase in risk.

Unfortunately, it doesn't stop there. The move away from milk and other dairy products towards soft drinks and fruit juices means, firstly, that we don't take in enough calcium. In fizzy drinks, there's a substance known as phosphoric acid – which some of the cleverer cola companies call food acid – that basically strips the calcium out of your bones. Thus, we're seeing marked increases in osteoporosis, especially in people who consume excessive amounts of soft drink. One study showed that teenagers who consume a cola-based drink on a daily basis have a seven times higher rate of bone fracture, and those who consume standard soft drinks have a rate five times higher.

The Paleolithic principle

This is very straightforward. If you can kill it and eat it straight away or grow it in your backyard, it's good for you, and after that all bets are off. Basically, what I'm saying is to eat less food and eat more naturally. We were not designed to put all this synthetic rubbish through our body. We were designed for natural foods such as fish, meat, eggs, dairy and, most importantly, vegetables. Fruits and vegetables should be the staple for all of us and the Walker-suggested dose is two or three pieces of fruit and three to five standard servings of vegetables per day (a serving of vegetables for example is half a carrot). That might sound pretty easy, but if it is, how come only 10 per cent of modern society takes in this amount of fruit and vegetables?

At this point I need to mention the whole concept of fat. From the scientific evidence, I strongly believe that saturated fats found in meat, dairy, and other foods such as coconuts and coconut oil, are neutral, i.e. they do not hurt nor do they help. The monounsaturated fats, such as found in olive oil and avocado, and the omega 3 fats, such as found in fish and nuts, are positively beneficial to the body and should be encouraged.

Body typing

One of the major themes of my book *Diets Don't Work* is that one size does not fit all. This book talks about the fact that we have four basic body shapes for women and one less for men. It gives you a simple guide as to what your particular body shape is and how you should eat more towards that body shape for weight loss and energy maintenance. The book also supplies a number of eating plans which will suit your body shape.

The 19 out of 21 rule

The final aspect of nutrition is what I call the Walker 19 out of 21 rule. For 19 meals each week you should follow the program; the other two you should do what you like. I don't believe any of us should be sentenced to a way of eating all of the time and if you really enjoy particular types of food that you know are not that good for you, see them as an occasional treat.

3. Exercise And Movement

The second-best drug on the planet is exercise. My suggested dose is three to five hours of exercise per week where you achieve that hot, short of breath stage. If you take your age away from 220, this is your predicted maximum heart rate. I suggest you try to get to 60 to 70 per cent of your predicted maximum heart rate. You don't need to actually take your pulse, you just need to know when you are a touch short of breath and starting to feel hot, because this is at about the right percentage of your predicted maximum.

Not only do we need to do three to five hours of exercise per week, we should also see everything we do as an opportunity for movement – move, move and move, as much as you can. One of the big problems in modern society is that usually (unless you're a professional sportsperson), the more successful you are, the more time you spend sitting at a desk. The majority of physical jobs tend to be the least paid jobs and many people can spend most of the day in a very stationary position. Another good idea is to purchase a pedometer and measure your number of steps – you should be trying to achieve around 10,000 steps every day. Make a conscious effort to park further away from your destination. Always take the stairs rather than the escalator.

At least three hours of exercise per week reduces your risk for heart disease, cancer and Alzheimer's disease by 30 per cent and osteoporosis by 50 per cent, as well as dropping your blood pressure by 15 to 20 mmHg.

Exercise – how much is enough?

The famous Australian swimmer Lisa Curry-Kenny has had her own battle with heart disease. Lisa is not a patient of mine and I am only relating what I have heard in the media, but it appears that she suffered a condition called viral myocarditis and, because of this, her heart developed a significant rhythm disturbance, necessitating the implantation of an implantable defibrillator. Many people are shocked that a fit athlete would suffer such a serious cardiac condition, as many people have the delusion that exercise makes you immortal.

Although I have already stressed the importance of regular exercise, this doesn't mean, however, that more exercise is better. We often hear of how high-performance athletes succumb to some premature illness, such as the one suffered by Ms Curry-Kenny.

In fact, unless you take a high-quality natural supplement program to negate the free radical effect of exercise, the rate of serious health problems may be increased by high-level exercise.

Many of us know the story of Jim Fixx, who wrote *The Complete Book of Running*. Mr Fixx suffered a heart attack at the age of 32; basically because he had a severe genetic problem which was never detected or treated and he was very unfit. He felt that running would be the answer and he began a very full running program, as well as writing that book. For 17 years, he ran many marathons and competed in many other races, but for about six weeks prior to his death was complaining of chest pain. Unfortunately, on the day of one of his races he felt very unwell but still competed, collapsing and dying during the race.

If you want to participate in high-performance athletics, you need to be prepared to have a supervised and full supplement program that will help negate the free radical effect. You will certainly develop a significant cardiovascular benefit from the exercise in most cases, but without that program, your immune system may become weakened and therefore set you up for a condition such as that suffered by Ms Curry-Kenny. She now has to spend the rest of her life with a reduced exercise program and an implantable defibrillator that will shock her heart back into a good rhythm if and when a bad heart rhythm occurs.

4. Quitting Addictions

It is impossible to be healthy and to have an addiction. If you smoke, you aren't healthy. If you drink too much alcohol, you aren't healthy, and if you use any illegal drugs whatsoever, you aren't healthy.

Really, the first step in stopping cigarettes – or any addiction – is a decision. In the case of smoking, once you make the firm decision that you really want to stop, you're well on the road to achieving this goal. Make your decision public. Tell your friends and relatives that you fully intend to stop and that you want their help. Really increase your desire to become a non-smoker and think of all the benefits to your life in doing so.

We now have quite good pharmacologic help in the form of nicotine patches, gums etc. There is also a drug called Zyban that was developed as an anti-depressant, which has shown some benefit in smoking cessation, although it is not good for a small proportion of the population who have suffered epilepsy. The most recent advance has been a drug called Champix that actually blocks the nicotine receptors in the brain and thus takes away your desire to smoke. Again, this is an excellent drug with minimum side effects apart from mild nausea, but should be avoided in people with strong psychiatric histories, as in this situation it may exacerbate a problem that is already present. There have also been some recent concerns about a cardiac risk in people using Champix, but the important point here is that the enormous risk of smoking far outweighs any minor risk of medication.

I tend to take smoking cessation one step further in my patients by putting the responsibility well and truly back onto them. You can talk to people about lung cancer, heart disease, chronic airways disease etc until you are blue in the face (or, more likely, until they are blue in the face if they keep smoking), but hitting someone at their intellect is not really the way to go. I often tell the story of a professor of respiratory medicine I worked for who spent all day telling people to stop smoking, but he himself had had bypass surgery twice and was still ducking out the back at lunchtime for a cigarette. Addiction is addiction.

THE DEATH OF IVAN

Ivan was a 57-year-old male who was still playing veteran's soccer. Four years previously, he suffered chest pain, assumed it was the start of a heart attack and drove himself to the hospital. Despite increasing chest pain, he stopped on the way to buy petrol and subsequently had his diagnosis confirmed – at the hospital, not the petrol station!

During the course of his admission, it was discovered that he had severe obstructions of his coronary arteries and it was suggested that he required coronary artery bypass grafting surgery. As is his undeniable right, Ivan refused the surgery or any pharmaceutical agents (including aspirin), preferring to follow a particular diet which he formulated himself. He took a bucket of natural supplements and continued to smoke.

Following this, he consulted with me (I hadn't met him before, either as a patient or on the soccer field) and was given the same advice he'd previously received – again, he declined. When I checked his heart on two occasions, the last a few months before his death, he continued to have severe lack of oxygen to his heart muscle despite having no symptoms whatsoever. I suggested on each occasion that he should stop smoking and avail himself of orthodox medical and surgical therapy for his disease, but once again he declined.

Recently, Ivan died suddenly, eating well but smoking to the day of his death. He had also continued to play veteran's soccer. The major point here is that had Ivan followed the medical advice given to him, it's almost certain that he'd be alive today. He was at very high risk for a cardiac event but ignored that risk, to his unfortunate premature demise.

Alcohol

Recently, two major issues have been raised regarding alcohol consumption. For many years I've been a strong supporter of the use of two small glasses of red wine per day as a cardiac preventative. However, recently the National Health and Medical Research Council (a scientific medical body in Australia) released its new guidelines regarding alcohol consumption. Safe consumption in males used to be said to be either four standard drinks or less per day and, for females, two standard drinks or less per day. These days, the new guidelines are saying it should be two standard drinks for everybody.

A report has also been recently released by the Cancer Institute of New South Wales, suggesting there is no safe level of alcohol consumption. This somewhat alarmist analysis suggests that there is a high risk from drinking just two glasses of any form of alcohol per day. They say that alcohol is particularly linked to cancer of the upper digestive and respiratory tracts, breast, colorectum, liver and stomach. There is not really much left when you think about this.

The report, entitled 'Alcohol as a Cause of Cancer', says the risk of cancer in the upper respiratory tract and upper digestive tract is increased by around 40 per cent, and the mouth and pharynx alone by 75 per cent. The breast cancer risk varies somewhere between 11 and 22 per cent higher in women who drink than in non-drinkers. Four drinks a day increases the risk of bowel cancer in males by 64 per cent. The finding goes on to quote many other less common cancers with a significant increase in risks.

Let me give my position on this. Firstly, I believe it is irresponsible for any doctor to encourage a patient to drink. The health benefits from consuming alcohol are not strong enough to justify suggesting this may be some form of medical treatment.

However, let me discuss two very important points in this debate. Firstly, the majority of the analyses about cancer and heart disease in relation to alcohol come from trials conducted in the USA. When one considers any therapy or toxin in isolation, one is practising very dangerous science. If a therapeutic trial is performed on a drug, all other aspects of that person's life are compared in what is known as a multivariate analysis. When a scientific trial considers alcohol consumption, many other aspects are not taken into consideration. For example, no-one could accuse the typical American diet of being a healthy one. It would be hard to imagine that there'd be any benefit from adding alcohol to this type of diet.

If you look at the majority of the trials out of the USA, there is at best a weak cardiovascular benefit from low-dose consumption of alcohol. But when you then consider the trials of a more healthy lifestyle, i.e. the Mediterranean, these consistently show that the combination of a Mediterranean style diet with a couple of glasses of red wine per day have a 50 per cent reduction in heart disease and cancer.

The point I'd like to make is that if you wish to have a couple of glasses of alcohol per day, my suggestion is to have somewhere between 125 and 250 ml of red wine most days, on a regular basis, but you must combine this with a healthy eating pattern and not live by the delusion that those couple of glasses will override eating bad food.

The second consideration I'd like to bring in here is the Nurses' Health Trials. These trials, which have been conducted in Harvard

University for over 25 years, have clearly showed around a 25 per cent increase in breast cancer even from low to moderate consumption of alcohol, unless the nurses supplemented with a multivitamin that had at least 400 mcg of folic acid, and then the breast cancer risk was negated.

Thus, it's my strong suggestion that if you enjoy one or two glasses of alcohol per day, make it red wine, combine it with a healthy diet and also take a multivitamin that has at least 400 mcg of folic acid. I believe this is the best way of continuing to enjoy your alcohol without running the risk of all the problems that have been quoted. If, however, you don't particularly enjoy drinking I certainly wouldn't suggest you take it up.

5. Mind Power

The most important drug in the world is a thing called happiness, peace and contentment. Living in our modern, complex world often leads to stresses and strains that can affect our ability to achieve this state. I believe there are five specific reasons why modern living causes such angst:

i. *Choice* – you might say that this is an unusual cause of stress and unhappiness, but the more choices you have to make, the more stresses this causes. This has been confirmed in numerous studies and many people talk about the benefits of having a simpler life that is uncluttered, with less choice.

ii. *Multi-skilling* – no longer can one person be expected to have an expertise in just one area. For instance, even with something as simple as sending emails and texting, we all have to become expert typists, and many people no longer have someone who'll send the emails for them or do the typing.

But really, there is no such thing as multi-skilling. It is better termed 'sequential processing'; in other words, if you're expected to do a number of different tasks at once, your brain files them in order, from most to least important.

iii. *Instant answers* – with mobile phones, emails and text messaging, many people are expected to be on 24 hour call and this is yet another cause of anxiety.

iv. *Change* – these days, you can't expect to have the same employment for the 30 to 40 years you're working and receive a gold watch at the end of your dedicated service. Many people will reinvent themselves five, six, seven times during their working life, and, although very good for the brain, being open to this change can cause stress.

v. *Litigation* – yes, the lawyers don't get out of this lightly. The threat of litigation in our modern world is increasing. I know that, in my job, there are not too many people who have not been sued by a patient for some reason.

Unrelated to the above five causes is a major global issue – overpopulation. Overpopulation and overcrowding, especially in our major cities, is a significant cause of stress. Also, despite excess people, factors such as social isolation and loneliness can contribute to significant problems.

Despite all of these issues, it's my firm belief that achieving peace, contentment and happiness is an internal, rather than an external, phenomenon. In my book *The Life Factor*, I detail extensively how stress arises and how we can manage all of the issues I've mentioned.

One of the features of that book is my five mind tonics, which are:

i. *Control* – we should see ourselves as an active participator in life. You should take the responsibility for the only thing you can take responsibility for, i.e. you. It is no-one else's job to make you happy: that is your job.

ii. *Commitment* – we should have a commitment to living now and to being emotionally up to date. We should not practise 'woundology'. Woundology is wearing an emotional trauma from earlier in your life on your sleeve and maintaining the wound, rather than practising the most important method of healing and becoming healthy, which is forgiveness. Once you forgive someone and move on in your life, then you can heal your wounds. If you maintain the hurt, you will not improve.

iii. *Challenge* – you should see a challenge every day in living life. You should see each situation as a test. Every interaction you have with any human being, no matter how insignificant it may seem to you, is a test of what sort of person you are.

iv. *Connectedness* – we should try to achieve a sense of belonging to the community and to people as a whole. Connectedness means feeling loved, supported and having that connection with other people. Again, this is not their job, this is your job.

v. *Capacity* – John Lennon once said that life is what happens while you're busy making other plans, and we should develop a capacity to deal with the unexpected, the uninvited and the unimaginable. There are many traumatic events in life, but it's how you deal with them that's important, and it's vital you develop the capacity to deal with these issues.

CHAPTER 10

Health by decades

❁ *'A journey of 1000 steps begins with a single step'* – Confucius

Most people would agree that a major goal of ours should be to live a long and healthy life. This all sounds very laudable but it's surprising and alarming how many people don't achieve this goal. I'd suggest that the majority fall well short of this aim and that, although many people survive to their late 70s or early 80s, they don't survive that well.

This fellow goes to the doctor and says, 'I want to live until I'm 100.' So the doctor says, 'Do you smoke?' 'No,' says the man. 'Do you drink?' 'Occasionally, but not very much,' replies the man. 'Do you overeat?' 'No, I'm normal body weight.' 'Do you exercise regularly?' 'Yes, somewhere between three to five hours every week.' 'Do you go out with wild women?' 'No, of course I don't, I've been married for well over 40 years.' The doctor looks at the patient and says, 'Well, what do you want to live to 100 for?'

I believe we should introduce health consciousness at a very early age. Fortunately, these days there are many, very well researched educational programs introduced even at the preschool level. Unfortunately, hormones typically kick in in the early teens and that's where the problem starts. These hormones are closely linked to rebellious and risk-taking behaviour, which often coincide with the development of some rather bad health habits. Poor eating and sleeping habits, coupled with the introduction of both legal and illegal drugs in the late teens and early 20s, is fairly typical in our modern era. The younger person's brain is wired for this type of behaviour and many people in their 20s think they are bullet proof.

To bombard this age group with sound health advice usually falls on deaf ears. Despite the numerous TV commercials about binge drinking, speeding or not smoking, we still see alarming rates of cigarette consumption and alcohol-related trauma, while the highest death rate from motor vehicle accidents is certainly in this age group.

For preventative health messages to be effective, I think it's more appropriate for this information to be individualised to particular age groups. So I've developed a concept of health by decades. For each decade, I'll cover what I believe to be the most important area of focus. In no way am I suggesting that this is all that is necessary, but as the Chinese philosopher Confucius stated (and he told me he was delighted to be quoted in my book), the small steps lead to the bigger steps.

Decade up to age 30

EXERCISE

From an early age, I believe it's vital to develop and maintain a lifelong exercise habit. I've already mentioned the enormous benefits of regular exercise in reducing the risk of all forms of vascular disease, cancer, diabetes and osteoporosis.

I believe that Carl Jung is the greatest psychiatrist ever, and he came up with an interesting concept called the 'archetypical stages of aging'. I've modified this somewhat, but interestingly it does coincide with the stages of health by decades.

The first stage of life is that of rapid learning, acquiring language skills as an infant etc. You learn language and additional life skills from your parents (hopefully), as well as from role models such as teachers. These skills typically include a vast array of important health tips and advice to keep you living well into your later years.

As I've suggested, all that flies out the window in your teens and early 20s, which I call the stage of 'Looks'.

Exercise should be highlighted as a key health point for teenagers and young adults. Young men usually don't go to the gym to maintain good health practices; they basically just want their bodies to look good and buffed. Similarly, young women don't avoid fast food for health reasons (if, in fact, they do avoid it) – their motivation is to avoid putting on weight. For the same reason, they go to the gym.

It's also up to the age of 30 that the human body is at its most supple. From 18 to 30, the muscles and joints, along with the vascular system, are at their optimal level and that's why most high-performance athletes are in this age group. I'm always amused (and for someone much older like me, somewhat disturbed) when I hear a 34-year-old sportsman being referred to as the veteran of the team!

So, start and maintain a lifelong exercise program during this decade.

Decade age 30 to 40

QUIT ADDICTIONS

Although learning and looks are still important, it is typically at this time that your position in life is being established. Whether this is your occupation, your emotional partnerships or another vital component, you have moved into what Jung called the archetype of competition. To win, you must be at the top of your game. You want to be the best at work, the best partner and the best performer, but there's a problem.

The bad habits you may have developed in the earlier decades are now starting to take effect. You're not recovering from that weekend binge anywhere near as well as you did a decade before. That 10- to 15-year smoking habit is now giving you a rather distasteful cough and you're much more short of breath running around the field playing your weekend sports.

In no way am I suggesting anyone should cultivate addictive behaviours at any age, but if you have, start thinking about removing these from your life before they have devastating health effects.

As I've said, one in five people carry the gene for nicotine addiction and it's probably close to one in 20 for alcoholism. If you're highly addicted to either of these drugs and are finding it very difficult to kick the habit, there are many health professionals with strong expertise in this area who can help.

I see quitting an addiction as a major personal achievement. I'd strongly suggest using any method possible that works for you.

John's story

John is a patient of mine who is a self-confessed alcoholic. A number of years ago, he realised that his alcoholism was destroying his life and joined Alcoholics Anonymous. This has been an enormous help to him and he's been free of alcohol since.

John has an extraordinary coping mechanism that allows him to stay away from the grog. This is his rather marvellous sense of humour. He often sends me a report on his AA meetings with an extremely humorous twist, or just makes some very astute and hilarious comment on life in general. Humour certainly works for John and I must say I find humour a vital part of my life as well.

Trent's story

Trent was in his late 30s and came to see me because he was suffering palpitations and his blood pressure was rising. On further questioning, he told me he ran his own business and earned around $5000 a week. However, he did have an obvious cause for his health issues – an addiction to free-base cocaine, otherwise known as crack. He'd used crack once a week for the last 10 years and it was costing him $1000 per week to maintain this habit.

I find that appealing to someone's head is of absolutely no value in getting them to lose an addictive habit. Telling him about the heart-attack, stroke and sudden-death rate amongst cocaine and crack users would really have been a waste of time. Crack is a highly addictive drug and one needs highly effective mechanisms to get people away from this dreadful plague.

On further questioning, I found that Trent's father had died in his early 40s of heart disease; hence his concern over the palpitations and his rising blood pressure.

Trent lived with his mother and was very close to her. I said to him, 'I want you to imagine a coffin in a church with your dead body in it. I want you to imagine your mother sitting in the front row crying uncontrollably, having her heart broken for the second time in her life. Do you have a right to do that to her? When you call by your dealer on the weekend, get that picture in your mind and see whether you still want to use the crack.'

The following week, Trent came back to see me and to thank me. For the first time in 10 years, he hadn't used the drug. The next day he didn't suffer palpitations and his blood pressure was entirely normal.

I haven't heard from Trent since and he may have gone back to the crack, or he may not have. The point is that if he could do it once, he could certainly do it again and do it permanently. It's all about making a decision.

In this situation, I talk about my 'Five Point Power Program'. 1. Make the decision; 2. Interrupt the road blocks; 3. Create a new program; 4. Train the program; 5. Live the program.

1. Life is all about making decisions. Whether they're small or big, it is the quality of the decisions you make that determines the quality of your life. If something is really dragging you down, such as an addiction, you must make the decision that you really want to stop this. Not only do you declare to yourself that you want to stop this addiction, tell the people who love you and

make a public declaration of your desire to get rid of whatever it is you want to change.

2. Interrupt the road blocks. Often addictions are associated with other psychological cues. For example, I had one patient who lived over the road from the Melbourne zoo and from her terrace she could look across and see the animals. She'd really look forward to coming home after a busy day's work, sitting out on her balcony watching the animals and having a cigarette. This psychological association made it almost impossible for her to stop smoking.

    I told her that she wasn't to smoke on the balcony anymore and, soon after, she lost the desire to smoke, as she certainly didn't need to smoke at all during the day at work. You must look at what patterns are stopping you from losing your addiction and get rid of them.

3. Create a new program. If you have an addiction, stopping this addiction does leave a hole in your life.

Allan's story

Around 15 years ago, I saw Allan as a patient. He had the most severe cardiomyopathy I've ever seen. When I performed an ultrasound of his heart, his heart walls were almost not moving. He had around 20 litres of extra fluid in his body because the heart wasn't pumping properly, and I told him and his wife that if he didn't stop drinking immediately, he'd be dead within the next few weeks.

Allan was a wharfie who used to arrive at work around 8 am, then wander over to the pub at about 10 o'clock and start drinking.

He'd consistently have 15 to 20 schooners every day and this was the cause of his severe dilative cardiomyopathy. Alcohol is a cellular poison and can certainly poison the heart, especially at this dose.

I told Allan that he was far too sick to continue working, so I interrupted his road blocks, i.e. drinking with his mates. The major issue here was that if you take 15 to 20 schooners out of someone's daily routine, it leaves a huge hole. To my enormous surprise, Allan filled this hole by developing an interest in ancient Egypt and became an amateur Egyptologist. He read as many books as he possibly could and attended many courses about the country and its history.

He then put all of the money he wasn't spending on beer into an account and saved this up. By the end of the year he'd accumulated enough to pay for a trip for himself and his lovely wife to visit the pyramids.

Over the past 15 years, Allan has remained a very faithful and valued patient of mine. A few years back, he came into my practice with a picture. He said to me, 'Ross, I want you to see a picture of my grandson Jake. Without you I wouldn't be enjoying him right now.' I said, 'No, Allan, without your extraordinary decision and life-changing habits, you wouldn't be here enjoying your life.' It was really his strength and innovation, not my advice, which allowed him to return to good health.

His heart has remained normal over the years, with only some minor issues that I've dealt with, and he has really enjoyed his life since making that incredible change.

4. Condition the habit. It takes at least a month of very hard discipline before a habit becomes ingrained; some people say even longer. It is really important that you bring in that discipline.

5. Live the program. Twelve-week courses or diets don't work because they are finite. Any health innovation has to be lifelong.

Decade age 40 to 50

FOOD FOR THOUGHT

One of the major themes of this book is the unfortunate fact that our body was only designed to function optimally until around age 40. A key feature here is metabolic slowing. As our metabolic processes become affected by all the mechanisms mentioned in the previous chapters, our metabolic efficiency slows. As our fat storage mechanisms lose their ability to process and distribute fat for fuel, the fat storage areas quickly become overloaded and, you guessed it, the fat accumulates.

In females, it accumulates especially around the backside and upper thighs, but while this doesn't look good, it doesn't actually harm the body. Dangerous fat accumulates in two main areas. The worst is belly fat. Belly fat isn't just an ugly lump of lard, it's also a marker for fat in more serious sites, such as the vital organs and the arteries.

Belly fat itself is an inflammatory organ as well, switching on the immune system. This fat is also a reservoir for toxic chemicals. I'll highlight in the chapter on environmental health the added danger of the accumulation of synthetic chemicals in abnormal fat and the health risks posed by this.

All of the above makes the immune system work overtime, contributing to many chronic diseases.

The other site of dangerous fat accumulation is around the throat.

Fat around this area is a major factor in the generation of sleep apnoea, which I covered in the chapter on fatigue.

So, I see the decade between 40 and 50 as the time when we should be focusing on our eating habits. The best advice here, as per the last chapter, is to eat less. It is this decade where you really start to notice the build-up of belly fat and, unless you start changing your food intake, I can assure you this won't stop.

I see this as the time of the role model. Typically, this decade sees people being firmly established in their careers with responsible positions. They have had enough experience to be able to teach and influence younger people coming through the ranks.

They are also role models for the most important people in their life – their family. Children, especially, are emotional and mental sponges. If their parents demonstrate and display healthy and responsible behaviour, this is usually seen and adopted by their children.

Of course, there will be rebellious years but I'd venture to say that by the time young adults are emerging from their late 20s to early 30s, the deeper aspects of parental influence are taking their effect. So I'd strongly suggest you constantly examine your own behaviour, as it not only affects your own health and quality of life but also that of your children.

Decade age 50 to 60

TAKE THE TEST

Although I believe every visit to your doctor should be an opportunity for health screening, it's important to have relatively simple checks starting in your 40s. But the big league, serious assessments should start during this decade. Let me make an important point that can't be emphasised enough. All your common diseases have their origins in your childhood, teens and early adulthood, but typically become manifest after age 50.

Our biggest killer, atherosclerosis, can often start in utero. At this point I'd like to introduce the concept of early vascular priming.

Hertfordshire Heart Study

Hertfordshire is the county immediately to the north of London. The Hertfordshire Heart Study followed the health patterns of around 5600 men born in the county between 1911 and 1930. They found three very interesting factors that influenced the risk of these men for coronary artery disease. Number one, low birth weight; number two, an inability to double their birth weight by one year old; number three, breastfeeding beyond 12 months.

All three factors, but especially low birth weight, were associated with a marked increase in heart disease risk. The theory is that malnourishment during pregnancy and for the first 12 months leads to immaturity in the blood vessels and a degree of mal-development. This commonly occurs in lower socioeconomic groups, who often have poorer eating habits. Once these young children were exposed to (often) excess calories with energy-dense but nutrient-poor foods, their immature, poorly developed blood vessels weren't strong enough to withstand this assault, and thus it was very easy for the fat to accumulate in the walls of their arteries at a very young age.

So, using the example of our most common disease process, atherosclerosis occurs very early on in your life and builds up over decades to eventually rupture into the channel of the blood vessels, blocking the arteries, leading to heart attack, stroke and sudden death.

However, it does usually take decades for this to occur. So if you don't have a rampant family history of heart disease (typically occurring before age 60 in first-degree relatives, i.e. parents, grandparents or siblings), or none of the other major risk factors for heart disease, age 50 is a good time to start screening.

Pre-conception, though, is a good time for your parents to start thinking about your health. Unfortunately, poor decisions and lifestyle behaviour on the part of your parents may impact on your health for decades to come. So, age 50 is also a very good time to be screened for the following common illnesses (see the Appendix for the appropriate tests):

1. Cardiovascular assessment, including diabetic screening and Alzheimer's disease for those with a family history;
2. Common cancers – prostate, bowel, breast, melanoma, lung for current and former smokers;
3. Osteoporosis.

Although I'm a great advocate and believer in screening, it's important to make the point strongly that there is no test in medicine that is 100 per cent accurate. I introduced coronary calcium scoring using CT technology into Australia in the late-90s, but while this is the most accurate screening test for heart-attack risk, as I've said, like all tests it isn't 100 per cent accurate. I occasionally see people who have heart attacks with zero scores, but there is no doubt that from the hundreds of thousands of people who've been screened and benefited from this technology, *the higher the score, the higher your risk.*

Screening for any condition is purely an indication of disease potential. Mammography is not always right – it sometimes over-diagnoses a cancer and sometimes misses a cancer. This is the nature of the disease and the nature of the test.

Now, this is a major point: symptoms always override test results. If you have a symptom, it always needs to be checked. If your calcium score was zero but six months later you start to experience chest pain, especially with exertion or stress, it is angina until proven otherwise. These symptoms do necessitate a rather urgent stress echo cardiogram.

A breast lump needs careful evaluation. Any gastrointestinal bleeding or change in bowel habits need a thorough gastrointestinal work-up.

In a simple sentence: don't ignore symptoms!

Decades 60 onwards

RECHARGE YOUR BRAIN

Sixty and beyond is typically the time we start slowing down. As our stress levels (hopefully) reduce, unfortunately often our need to think and stay active in body and mind may start to decline.

So I call this period in our life the age of the mind. This is where we should be taking active steps to keep the mind as sharp as possible. If you haven't already done so, I'd strongly suggest reading the superb book by Dr Norman Doidge, *The Brain that Changes Itself.* I believe this is one of the best summaries on the topic of maintaining mental sharpness. There is no point living to 100 if you can't remember why you're doing so!

Jung stated that as we lived beyond 50, we moved into the stage of the Sage. I believe this is best summarised as the age of wisdom and peace. As I've stated, the ultimate aim of life is to achieve peace, happiness and contentment, but unfortunately there are still a number of people who don't seem to get it (I mean, both understand this point and achieve it).

After 50, we should be imparting wisdom, not just to ourselves but to those around us. The principles of mentoring and teaching are so important here. Passing on that wisdom to the younger generations, both at work and to our families, is vital and a necessary part of a functioning society.

Although I've approached this chapter in decades, I'm making the point that all of these health suggestions are vital. Once you've mastered one suggestion, this should stay with you for the rest of your life.

I strongly recommend you see every day as a life improvement strategy. How can you be better at everything you do? Cultivate the observer inside you. The observer is that watcher inside who non-judgementally monitors your behaviour, gives advice and reminds you of your true values and desires.

The more effort you put into assessing, changing and then maintaining good life behaviours, the less effort the medical profession will need to put in to undo any damage done.

PART II

CHAPTER 11

The five stages of health

I started medical school in 1974. I'd developed a desire to be a doctor from my mid-teens, sparked by a keen interest in science and mathematics. I had no idea what a career in medicine would entail.

My mother (bless her departed soul) told me I was too lazy to be a doctor and encouraged me to be a maths teacher. I apologise to all those hardworking maths teachers out there. My mother's strong point was certainly not career advice.

Having been trained in and practised conventional medicine since that time, I'm well aware of the power and life-changing ability of orthodox therapies to profoundly affect the course of someone's health and life, usually in a positive way.

Medicine does work. However, I believe the problem is that doctors and many patients put too much faith in this form of healing. In fact, orthodox or 'mechanical' health strategies hardly ever heal.

Orthodox medicine has powerful methods to combat symptoms, remove diseases (typically with a scalpel) and alter the course of a variety of sometimes rather nasty conditions. But it hardly ever cures.

Healing implies something much more profound. If you ask most conventional doctors why people develop diseases, you'll get answers such as genetics, risk factors, other environmental issues or, at times, pure bad luck. There will be no discussion of mind, health and body interaction, energy medicine, or any suggestion to explore healing techniques outside the conventional approach.

As I've said, we live in a physical world that has flaws, which is precisely why we are here in the first place. But those flaws have the downsides that nothing works perfectly and nothing lasts forever.

You may believe that life has no inherent purpose and we are purely evolving members of the food chain or, alternatively, that there is a much deeper purpose (as I believe). Regardless of your beliefs, you want to ensure that you have quality health, quality life and, with that, as much longevity as you can muster.

I therefore believe that we should also see every day as part of our healing process. Healing from what, you may ask. Take your pick. I think it would be hard to find anyone who has not been traumatised by something, not suffered some illness, or who is not at risk for some condition as their life progresses.

Once you start becoming aware of your own mortality (which usually starts after age 30, but as people are becoming more educated, this is occurring earlier with some), you would like strategies to achieve these important goals. So I believe to maintain true health, with both a quality of life and longevity, you need to involve yourself at each of the five stages of health:

1. **Body Health** – doctors are important and I believe it is vital to have a long-term relationship with a trusted physician.

2. **Environmental** – both our microcosmic environment (the internal environment of the body) and macrocosmic environment (the external environment, the community and the world as a whole) are breeding grounds for all manner of subtle and not-so-subtle health problems. There is no point pursuing health and healing if you exist in a toxic micro- or macrocosmic environment.

3. **Genetic** – it is your genes that load the gun and your environment that pulls the trigger. You may live a pristine life but lousy genes can still take you off the planet early. This highlights the vital importance of screening.

   In a recent test, one of my medical colleagues in her 60s had a calcium score of her coronary arteries. Anything above 400 is serious; hers was in the 800s. This woman is an expert in nutritional medicine, doesn't have an ounce of body fat and is a non-smoker, but she leads the life of a stressed general practitioner.

   She has also picked the wrong relatives with numerous members of her family suffering heart disease at an early age. Had she been a prolific self-abuser, she may have suffered heart disease a decade earlier. As it is, she still hasn't had a heart event, so we need to get stuck into reversing her disease. Thus, the importance of screening.

4. **Emotional** – you can't stand your partner, your kids are dropouts and on drugs, your job is super-stressful and, just to temporarily interrupt things, you decide to have a heart attack. After that's been treated, you go back to your situation. Nothing changes!

One of the reasons people don't heal is that they can't, won't, or aren't advised to change their situation. Life's problems, illnesses and traumas tend to have many factors. There is hardly ever one cause for a health issue, or for a problem you might have with others or within yourself. One aspect that can be changed is your situation or, more appropriately, your attitude to your situation.

I often tell my patients to go into any situation or interaction with a person with the attitude, 'I'm not going to give you the power to cause my heart attack or stroke.' There is this wonderful saying, 'Choose peace over this.' In many ways, peace is a moment-by-moment decision.

5. **Mind Health** – many people are unhappy because of their situation, the circumstances of their life. They are in a bad marriage, they have poor relationships with their children, many people feel socially isolated and a number of people don't enjoy their job and dislike their boss and co-workers.

    Although these may all be legitimate concerns, there is another way of looking at your life. Regardless of your religious beliefs, I still believe you should see every situation, every trauma, every interaction with every living being as symbolic. What is the underlying meaning? What is this experience trying to teach you?

    All we have in life is the moment. Life is all about this moment-by-moment management of your energy circuits. I have no scientific proof that we have energy centres in our body. They may or may not exist, so the section later in the book is pure hypothesis.

But I will argue that every moment occurs as part of a field of energy that we have control over. The problem is that we are working with our flawed biology. The DNA that makes us human also makes us flawed.

This is not just a biological structure – it also responds to a variety of energetic and environmental stimuli that it receives on a moment-by-moment basis.

We certainly need to develop better medicines, nutraceuticals, surgeries and other forms of mechanical therapies to combat the varying diseases that wreak havoc in the body. But we also need to cultivate better techniques to manage these energy centres, known by the ancient Indian gurus as 'chakras'. Later, I'll present the energy centre theory and also suggest practical steps in how to rebalance and manage your energy imbalances.

Health is a life process, a daily effort – I'd even venture to say that it's one of our major life purposes. If you follow and work through the five stages of health, you're well on your way not only to longevity, but quality health and quality life.

CHAPTER 12

Stage 1 – body health

In 1900, the average life expectancy was 47 years. At the time, only one person in 25 survived to the age of 60. One hundred years later, life expectancy has sky rocketed to around 80. Admittedly, this is very variable, with African countries typically rating somewhere between 40 and 50, although infant survival rates certainly skew the results down in underprivileged countries.

There is no doubt that improved living standards have raised the bar, but there is also an enormous contribution from modern medicine. The 20th century saw amazing advances in therapeutics, diagnostics and surgical techniques. Operations including anaesthesia have become sophisticated to a point where minimally invasive techniques, robotics and catheter-based procedures have replaced many of the archaic strategies of yesteryear.

All of the extraordinary advances in medicine are a result of painstaking research and brilliant medical scientists from all over the world. Science has always demanded rigorous testing and solid proof before introducing new advances into everyday practice.

It is these high standards that have ensured the level of safety of the vast majority of medical therapies and procedures. But things still go wrong – why? Because nothing is perfect. Doctors are flawed human beings. Nurses don't always check the patient correctly and administrative paperwork often goes astray and is incorrect. Medical therapies have the potential for side effects and don't always work. Surgical procedures can be complicated by bleeding, infection and human error at many levels, not to mention all of the hospital-acquired issues that may occur, including the excess of bureaucracy that has now infected most hospital systems.

However, don't forget the proven advances. With the advent of x-rays, which have evolved into the very sophisticated CT scanners and the non-x-ray MRIs, medical diagnosis and early detection has taken medical services to a new level. Antibiotics, introduced in the 1940s, revolutionised the practice of medicine. Before they became widely available, it wasn't uncommon for people – including children, teenagers and young adults – to die from pneumonia, urinary tract infections and a whole host of other bacterial infections. Millions of lives have been saved over the past 70 years because of the judicious use of antibiotics.

Of course, antibiotic overuse has led to resistant organisms and, at times, very serious side effects, but antibiotics have saved many more lives than they've harmed. For some bizarre reason I don't understand, vaccinations are very divisive therapies. There is a strong anti-vaccination lobby who have very short memories. These people should take a walk through a cemetery and see all the children who died in the earlier part of last century from diphtheria, whooping cough, tetanus, polio and measles. Smallpox has been wiped off the face of the earth due to vaccination.

Because of many people being opposed to vaccination, we're seeing a recurrence of whooping cough. A four-week-old child on the north coast of New South Wales died recently, probably because her mother wasn't vaccinated against whooping cough – the transfer of antibodies from the parent would have prevented this unnecessary death.

The British researcher Dr Andrew Wakefield has recently been discredited for his flawed research suggesting a link between the MMR (measles, mumps, Rubella) vaccine and autism. Basically, there is no scientific evidence whatsoever to support his claims.

Advances in the management of acute heart disease have seen the reduction of death from this often lethal condition. Before I entered medicine in the 1970s, the in-hospital death rate from heart attack was around 30 per cent. It is now below 3 per cent. (Of course, I'm not suggesting it's because I entered medicine.)

Although not as dramatic, survival rates from many cancers have improved significantly and, with early detection from improved diagnostic capability, a number of people have been cured. I have no doubt that the next 10 years will see significant advances in the very early detection of cancers, more individualised diagnoses and targeted therapies that minimise the side effects of current chemotherapeutic approaches.

I've got cholesterol, doc!

In terms of modern medicine, the most prescribed drug in the world is Lipitor, used to lower cholesterol. Lipitor is from a group of drugs known as statins, which block the last step in cholesterol production in the liver.

I'd suggest that well over 99 per cent of the general public has no real understanding of the nuances of cholesterol, but unfortunately the same can probably be said for the medical profession. There are so many misconceptions about cholesterol that I could devote an entire book to how it should be approached and managed, but I doubt this would be a best-seller.

I recently had a patient come to see me who was told by their GP that if they didn't take a particular statin drug to lower their cholesterol, they'd probably die. Suffice to say, I spend a significant proportion of my week dealing with matters cholesterol, so I'll try my best to summarise these issues briefly.

Firstly, and most importantly, if I took all of the cholesterol out of your body, you'd be dead within 24 hours. Cholesterol is a vital substance, which is a major building block to many hormones and an important component of every cell wall. Cholesterol is not a killer, nor is it the cause of heart disease. Nor, in most cases, do eggs or shellfish have a particularly strong effect on raising your cholesterol. Also, just because your cholesterol is elevated does not automatically mean that the fat is spilling into your arterial wall and setting you up for heart disease. Too many people in the medical profession treat cholesterol and not cardiovascular risk, but more of that later.

It's important to realise that the majority of cholesterol is made in your liver and does not come from dietary sources. The ratio would be about 70 to 30 per cent. It's also very important to realise that it is more dietary trans fatty acids and, to a lesser extent, saturated fat, along with processed carbohydrates, which raise serum cholesterol, and not dietary cholesterol, such as eggs and shellfish.

In fact, the best way to reduce your cholesterol level by dietary means is to cut down on your caloric intake, eat healthily, as I described earlier, and increase your exercise.

Moving further ahead to the contribution of cholesterol to heart disease, there's no doubt that there is an association, but it is not a definite one-on-one relationship. Interestingly, around 30 per cent of people who have heart disease have completely normal cholesterol levels. It is not just a matter of looking at total cholesterol levels but also at the cholesterol/HDL (good cholesterol) ratio, which ideally should be less than 3.5. So, if your total cholesterol is 7.0 but your HDL cholesterol is 2.0, your ratio is 3.5, which is ideal. I don't know how many times I see doctors, including cardiologists, treating these sorts of cholesterol levels in people who have no other risk factors for heart disease. There isn't one shred of evidence that using a pill for this situation will prolong your life at all.

The reality is that we should be treating cardiovascular risk and not cholesterol levels.

Now we come to a discussion of statin drugs. Statins have been around for over 20 years and, in fact, the only mortality benefit from statins has been seen in middle-aged males either with a proven history of heart disease or deemed to be at very high risk for heart disease because of multiple risk factors. There has never been any mortality benefit seen in females, low-risk males or the elderly.

There is, however, no doubt that if you commence a statin agent you reduce risk for a heart attack by around 20 to 30 per cent. The average middle-aged male is at about a 1 per cent per year risk for a cardiac event. The average middle-aged female is probably around a

0.5 per cent risk until around 10 years after the menopause, when her risk approaches that of a male. Using this simple formula it means that the average 55-year-old male or 65-year-old female is at about a 10 per cent 10-year risk for a heart attack, regardless of any other factors.

Once you start bringing in other aspects, such as high cholesterol, high blood pressure, cigarette smoking and diabetes, you increase the risk, and the presence of all four major risk factors with a family history in this age group probably gives you around a 50 per cent 10-year risk. Taking this argument further, using a statin drug to lower your cholesterol in this setting will reduce your risk by 20 per cent. Therefore, if you take a statin drug when you are at high risk, your risk goes from 50 per cent down to 40 per cent over 10 years.

If I was at a 50 per cent risk over 10 years for some form of heart disease, I would definitely take a statin to reduce my absolute risk by 10 per cent. However, I would certainly not put a strong synthetic agent with all of its inherent side effects through my system for a 10-year period for a small reduction in risk.

If your risk is only 10 per cent over 10 years and you take a statin drug, you again drop your risk by 20 per cent, which brings you down to 8 per cent. When you really look at the numbers the benefits are not that great, but still doctors persist in the widespread use of statins, even in people who are deemed at low risk for long-term events. If I was only deemed to be at a 10 per cent risk by risk factor analysis, thus reducing my absolute risk by only 2 per cent by taking a statin, I certainly wouldn't.

More significantly, achieving your ideal body weight, improving your diet by eating better quality food and less of it, having a regular exercise habit four or five times a week, quitting any addictions, and learning to enjoy your life by improving your relationships with people and developing a positive, happy outlook, will overall reduce your risk for any disease by 70 per cent. Thus, the combination of lifestyle factors and statins will give you a 90 per cent reduction in risk.

So if you start off with a 50 per cent risk over 10 years, you reduce your risk to 5 per cent, which is less than the average person of the same age. And if your risk is only 10 per cent and you bring in the lifestyle modification without the statins, the 70 per cent reduction drops your risk down to 3 per cent.

Swallowing any pharmaceutical agent doesn't give you a 100 per cent guarantee against developing a disease. Then again, neither does lifestyle modification. Medical treatment, whether it be lifestyle modification, pharmaceutical therapy or vitamin therapy, is about lowering and mini-mising risk, but there is no technique that will absolutely abolish it.

Regrettably, too many people, including members of the medical profession, believe that by swallowing a statin drug you abolish your risk for a disease. Nothing could be further from the truth, and even worse still is the concept that if you're swallowing a statin you really don't need to bother with lifestyle. Look at the numbers I've quoted above and you'll see the point I'm trying to make.

Unfortunately, there has been a strong misconception that I am against the use of pharmaceutical agents. I strongly support their appro-priate use, but I'm very much against the inappropriate use of drugs such as cholesterol-lowering agents for people who don't really need them. There is no doubt that if you've been deemed to be at high risk for heart disease or have already had a heart attack, bypass or a stent in your arteries, or a stroke or possibly even peripheral vascular disease, you definitely need assistance over and above lifestyle modification. This assistance is usually in the form of a statin drug, aspirin and some other medications.

It is my plea to the public and my colleagues that we adopt a more sensible approach to this subject, with a healthy debate on the issues, rather than making patients feeling guilty if they ask questions as to why they should take these drugs in the first place.

Over the years, a number of natural compounds have become available to lower cholesterol and been greeted with enormous enthusiasm by the complementary medical world, only to be treated with disdain or totally ignored by the vast majority of the medical profession.

From red rice extracts to substances derived from sugar cane, all have shown only minimal reductions in cholesterol. At best, you may see somewhere between a 10 to 15 per cent reduction in total cholesterol as opposed to a 30 to 40 per cent reduction seen with an average dose (10 to 20 mg) of Lipitor. A 10 to 15 per cent reduction in cholesterol is also seen with sensible diets, plant sterol-based margarines and certain specific foods such as nuts, olive oil and avocado.

Recently, major research has been published in peer-review journals about a new natural substance from bitter oranges grown in the Calabrian region of Italy. This product is being marketed under the name Bergamet, from Bergamot oranges, and it has been shown to reduce total cholesterol by around 30 per cent, LDL (bad cholesterol) by 38 per cent and triglycerides by up to 40 per cent, as well as increasing the HDL (good cholesterol) by up to 42 per cent. Bergamet also reduces blood sugar by somewhere between 20 and 30 per cent.

Warrick's story

Warrick is a 58-year-old diabetic with a waist circumference of 132 centimetres, cholesterol on statin therapy of 4.8 mm/L and a fasting blood sugar level of 7.7. He commenced Bergamet at a dose of 1000 mg a day (two capsules twice daily before meals) and after three months he'd lost 8 centimetres off his waist, his cholesterol had dropped from 4.8 down to 3.7, his blood sugar level had dropped from 7.7 to 4.1 and he had to stop one of his anti-diabetic pills because his sugar was dropping too low.

Not only has Bergamet been demonstrated to have these effects on important blood parameters, it has also been shown to prevent the progression of atherosclerosis in laboratory animals and improve blood vessel stiffness in human trials.

It is my firm opinion that Bergamet is:

1. an excellent solution for people experiencing significant side effects from statin drugs;
2. a viable addition to statin therapy for people experiencing minor statin side effects, i.e. add Bergamet to a reduced dose of statin;
3. an excellent solution for those with a strong aversion to taking pharmaceutical therapy;
4. excellent for those with a high cholesterol but no prior history of ischaemic heart disease (blockages in the coronary arteries), or deemed by non-invasive tests as being low risk.

For further information, I'd suggest you visit www.bergamet.com.

The major point here is that atherosclerosis occurs in all of us to some extent, once our cholesterol rises above 3 mmol/L and our systolic (top reading) blood pressure rises above 100 mm Hg. There aren't too many people wandering around in modern society with parameters below this level.

Thus, the lower you run your cholesterol and systolic blood pressure, the lower your atherosclerotic load and therefore the lower your risk for all forms of cardiovascular disease. If I thought statins were harmless, I'd take them myself. I certainly believe they're very effective in what they're supposed to be doing – lowering cholesterol – but I'm not convinced about their long-term safety, despite strong reassurances from the drug companies, who've made billions of dollars in sales of statin drugs.

There are a number of cardiologists all over the world who swallow statins every day, like a vitamin, because they are deluded into believing these drugs will offer them immortality. However, a recent report suggested that there is not enough evidence to recommend the widespread use of statins for people with no previous history of heart disease.

Over the years, there have been numerous claims by the complementary therapists regarding the ability of a variety of vitamins and herbal preparations to reduce blood pressure.

The vast majority are ineffective and some have a marginal effect.

Recently, an Australian company, Dr Red, has produced a commercial product from purple carrots. Independent research from the University of Southern Queensland has shown significant reductions in blood pressure, equivalent to a standard blood pressure pill.

Purple carrots are the ancient form of carrot which were in existence long before the more commonly consumed orange carrots. These carrots are rich in very strong phytochemicals known as anthocyanins. They have been studied in spontaneously hypertensive rats. No, I know what you're thinking. I'm not referring to a bunch of anally retentive rodents who are constantly worried about fluctuations in the stock market; I'm referring to rats who have been genetically primed to have high blood pressure.

You guessed it: the purple carrots dropped the blood pressure as efficiently as standard blood pressure pills prescribed by doctors. Preliminary human trials have demonstrated similar results.

The natural cholesterol-lowering substance Bergamet, which I've mentioned before, has also been shown to have a reasonable effect in dropping blood pressure to around the same level as the purple carrots.

SLEEP APNOEA

I can't leave the topic of non-pharmaceutical management of high blood pressure without a mention of this very common condition. Apart from the aforementioned forms of lifestyle indiscretions, sleep apnoea is the commonest cause for refractory hypertension.

So if you and your doctor are struggling to control your blood pressure, especially if you are waking unrefreshed, very tired and suffering daytime sleepiness, it's important you are investigated for sleep apnoea.

PHARMACEUTICAL THERAPY

Especially if you are over 50, managing your blood pressure is much more important than lowering cholesterol. I'm not denying the importance of cholesterol but I'm certainly stressing the importance of keeping your blood pressure controlled. Modern medicine has a vast array of very effective, safe medications to control blood pressure. As far as I'm concerned, the above lifestyle factors, management of sleep apnoea and any other trick you can muster are not negotiable and should be part of the regimen of anyone who is prone to hypertension.

But, if your blood pressure is still poorly controlled, you need to work with your doctor to find the right combination of medications to assist you in keeping your blood pressure at the right level.

At this point, I'd like to say that it is unacceptable for any doctor to prescribe any medication that causes long-term side effects. If I expect you to take a pill for the rest of your life, you must be comfortable taking that pill and it should not cause you any significant manner of side effects. There's a saying in medicine that it's hard to make a person with no symptoms feel better, but it's certainly quite easy to make them feel worse with modern therapeutics.

It is my strong belief that all pharmaceutical agents have the potential for side effects. Basically any pill can cause any side effect in any person. Thus, when someone comes to see me and is complaining of a new symptom, I always ask them about their medications and if the symptoms started soon after taking them. Then I blame the pill first and try to find an alternative approach to managing their condition.

For example, one of the most prescribed medications for high blood pressure is a set of drugs known as ACE inhibitors. Although these drugs are superb at managing blood pressure, 10 per cent of people who take them experience a dry cough which, at times, can be quite debilitating. If it's occasionally clearing your throat, I believe it is quite acceptable for the pill to induce this side effect. If, however, you're up all night coughing, there is no way you should be taking these medications.

An exhaustive analysis of the potential side effects of blood pressure drugs is certainly not within the scope of this book, but suffice to say if you have any new symptoms after taking medications always discuss this with your doctor.

I've already detailed the strategies for assessing and managing many of the common cancers. Over the next decade we'll see an explosion of targeted cancer diagnoses and therapies. Almost on a monthly basis, new genetic tests and specific anti-cancer antibodies and medications are trialled and assessed in major medical journals.

In all areas of orthodox medicine, i.e. mechanical health or body health, there are exciting new advances which are offering people much safer, more effective, less invasive therapies, allowing a much better chance for longer, quality lives.

With recent advances in genetic diagnoses, gene therapy and the variety of stem cell therapies now available, many diseases that destroyed quality of life and markedly reduced lifespan have now been treated when only supportive therapy was previously available.

As I've said, regardless of your attitude towards orthodox versus complementary medicine, my strong advice is that if you have significant medical problems, don't walk away from orthodox medicine. It has a proven evidence base with a long and successful track record. It should always be part of the treatment regimen in a person with serious medical problems – but it is not always enough.

CHAPTER 13

Stage 2 – environmental health

When I say the word environment, you probably think of the general state of the world, and concepts such as pollution, population and climate change. You may regard those individuals and – more likely – corporations that show little regard for the environment as environmental vandals, ripping down forests, utilising fossil fuels and spewing toxic waste into the atmosphere.

But anyone who avails themselves of the benefits of the modern world is an environmental vandal. Yes, we are all guilty and unfortunately we are all paying the price. Simply purchasing this book either in paper or the electronic version contributes in a small way to environmental disruption, although the value you'll get from reading it hopefully outweighs the detriment.

The bottom line is that, apart from the very small minority of people who live on this planet in a totally natural manner, humans are collectively environmental vandals.

Our increasing reliance on a whole host of subtle and not-so-subtle synthetic chemicals, along with electromagnetic radiation in increasingly man-made forms, is causing damage and illness both in the environment as a whole, and in our own personal environment. We are certainly being affected by these processes and these effects are almost certainly more serious than you'd imagine.

To begin with, I'd like to weigh in to the climate change debate. Let me make the analogy between this scenario and one of our major common killers. I believe that the argument between the climate change believers and the climate change sceptics detracts from the main issue. Personally, I think it is irrelevant whether there is or isn't climate change.

This is my argument. Our second most common killer in modern society is cancer. Cancer rapidly divides and multiplies, basically ripping the nutrients out of the host and spewing toxic by-products into the body. If there is a degree of change in the temperature in the body, this is a minor manifestation of a bigger issue, i.e. cancer.

The cancer on our planet is overpopulation. As a species, we are rapidly multiplying, ripping the raw materials or nutrients out of the earth and spewing toxic waste into the environment.

If there is a slight rise or drop in the temperature it doesn't really matter. Whether carbon or greenhouse gases effect global warming is the least of our concerns. The marked increase in synthetic chemicals and human-induced radiation is damaging the planet and the health of all living species, including ourselves.

It is not the carbon footprint of each and every individual that is the problem, it is the footprint in general. The planet cannot cope with its current human population, let alone the marked increases expected over the next few decades. I'm not giving the solution, I'm raising the point that we need to tackle the real problem, not the peripheral issue of whether or not climate change is taking place.

Almost every aspect of modern living is driven by the sun, from synthetic chemicals (typically derived from raw natural materials) to man-made electromagnetic radiation. Big business, in all its guises, would like us to believe that there is no significant detrimental effect on the body from our exposure to these, similar to the executives from cigarette companies who tried to argue that cigarettes were harmless.

Mind you, not all natural substances are harmless. A snake bite can kill you unless the anti-venom is close by! But with electromagnetic radiation and synthetic chemicals, there is a very simple principle. The bigger the dose, the longer the exposure and the more toxic the substance, the more acute and severe the effects on the individual. So, if a nuclear bomb explodes near you and the initial blast doesn't kill you, your chance of dying soon after from radiation poison is rather high. We have recently experienced the Japanese tsunami and the subsequent damage to the Fukushima nuclear power plant and all its potential serious health consequences.

But this then begs the question – what is the safe dose of a poison? My answer to this is zero. However, the argument from supporters of the use of electromagnetic radiation and synthetic chemicals is: what constitutes a poison and show me the evidence.

Firstly, let me consider the obvious, almost universally accepted poisons and then focus on the issues of electromagnetic radiation and synthetic chemicals.

Accepted toxins

1. *Food* – now hang on, we all need to eat! But almost everyone in modern society (and the author is definitely included in this) eats more than their body needs for a normally functioning metabolism.

   So, I would consider excessive calories a kind of poison that should be seen as part of environmental toxicity. Even more widespread is the HI factor. Professor Jennie Brand-Miller from the School of Nutrition at Sydney University pioneered the concept of the GI glycaemic index. Although I agree this is a vital aspect of managing the metabolic syndrome (the consequence of insulin resistance), I would suggest the HI factor is even more important.

   My friend, colleague and fellow health speaker on the professional speaking circuit, Dr John Tickell, pioneered this term. It stands for the Human Interference factor. Basically, how much have humans interfered with the food by the time it reaches your mouth? As I've mentioned previously, a simple principle here is that the more fiddling, the worse it is for you.

2. *Cigarettes* – forget about nicotine. This is the chemical in cigarettes that makes you addicted but it is the least toxic of the 48 serious poisons in cigarettes. With each cigarette you run the risk of either rupturing a fatty plaque in one of your arteries or inducing a lung cancer, and therefore there is only one answer here. At the risk of repeating myself, don't smoke.

3. *Alcohol* – any more than two standard drinks per day on a regular basis and you are putting your body at risk. Alcohol is a general cellular poison that wreaks havoc with every cell, especially your liver, heart and brain. It also raises your risk for diseases in all parts of your body.

4. *Illegal drugs* – any person who claims illegal drugs are harmless and should be made freely available has probably had their brain affected by illegal drugs.

Evidence emerges almost on a weekly basis demonstrating the health detriments from these substances. From the ability of marijuana to contribute to serious mental illnesses, to cocaine and related substances causing heart attacks, stroke and sudden death, these agents cause havoc across the globe. As I've mentioned, I believe the only reason they don't wreak more havoc is that they are expensive, illegal and hard to get.

It is not within the scope of this book to discuss the social and ethical issues of government-sponsored programs to administer drugs to registered addicts, or the enormous profits to bosses of drug cartels by the maintenance of the illegality of drugs.

Andrew is a 34-year-old man who had used cocaine intermittently over the previous 10 years. He went out to a friend's buck's party and had too much to drink and had a few lines of cocaine. The next day Andrew had a serious heart attack requiring a coronary stent but still scarred a significant proportion of his heart muscle.

Not everyone who uses cocaine will have a heart attack but the risks are so much higher and should be seen as a significant consequence of this dreadful drug.

5. *Obvious toxins* – nuclear fall-out. The serious health effects from excessive nuclear exposure from either the dropping of atomic bombs, controlled nuclear testing or serious accidents, such as Chernobyl or the more recent accident at the Fukushima nuclear facility, are not disputed.

6. *Chemical poisoning* – accidents such as the Union Carbide plant in Bhopal, India or large spills such as the *Exxon Valdez* cause significant health and environmental issues.

   Many local communities have been affected by being in the vicinity of large industrial plants which spill their toxic waste into the soil or the water supply.

7. *Infectious contamination* – we hear, all too often, about outbreaks of infections, typically in the water supply. Bugs ranging from giardia and cryptosporidium to the more serious cholera, typhoid and salmonella keep recurring all over the world.

Now to the major part of the chapter, the health detriments of electro-magnetic radiation and synthetic chemicals.

1. Electromagnetic radiation

Electromagnetic radiation (EMR) is both natural from the sun and, more typically, from man-made sources. It is divided into non-ionising and ionising. Non-ionising is EMR in the lower frequency range and includes power lines, TV and radio, radar, microwaves, mobile phones and towers, along with satellite dishes. The highest non-ionising frequencies include solar, light globes and radiant heaters, as well as visible light.

Ionising radiation includes ultra-violet light, x-rays, gamma rays from a variety of nuclear sources and cosmic radiation. For anyone interested in exploring the subject fully, I can recommend the excellent book by Lyn McLean, *The Force,* as well as *Dirty Electricity* by Donna Fisher.

Lyn McLean offers a superb summary of all the potential health issues related to non-ionising EMR. Rather than pure scare-mongering, Lyn provides practical solutions to minimise our exposure to EMR which, in reality, is inevitable if you choose to exist in the modern world. *The Force* presents a clear link between many common and serious health issues and the various sources of EMR. As with most toxins, the higher the dose and longer the length of exposure, the clearer the link to these conditions. From the available evidence, there appears to be a reasonably clear link between all forms of EMR and a variety of human cancers, Alzheimer's and other chronic neurodegenerative diseases such as motor neurone disease.

There is also disturbing evidence linking EMR and problems becoming pregnant and maintaining pregnancy, with contributions from male and female exposure to EMR. Again, if the foetus survives the pregnancy, there appears to be a link with birth defects and sudden infant death syndrome.

There is less strong evidence linking EMR, cardiovascular diseases and diabetes, as well as some suggestion of an EMR link to asthma and allergies. There is also the new EMR sensitivity syndrome which has a variety of symptoms rather similar to chronic fatigue syndrome.

I'd also like to make special mention of the relationship between mobile phone use and brain tumour. The well-respected brain surgeon Dr Charlie Teo has conducted research, along with his years of experience, showing a disturbing link between mobile phone use and a variety of brain tumours. The World Health Organization released the results of a trial at the start of 2010 suggesting a 30 per cent increase in the serious brain tumour malignant glioma in those who use mobile phones for half an hour per day for more than 10 years. As with cigarette smoking, there is generally a lag time before the health issues arise.

But here's the issue. Relatively short-term industry sponsored trials have not demonstrated any major health risk with the variety of forms of EMR. Strangely, the independent trials are the studies which demonstrate harm. To quote from *The Force*, 'Statements such as "that there is no evidence of risk" at levels of radiation below international standards are misleading and, of course, untrue. There is abundant evidence from hundreds of studies of risk from exposure levels below international standards. To reiterate: it's been shown to cause changes in cells and hormones consistent with cancer, reduce the protective effects of melatonin, create potent free radicals, trigger the release of heat shock proteins that cause cancer, reduce immunity and trigger allergic reaction, and it has been linked to genetic damage.'

In order to undermine these discoveries the phrase 'no consistent scientific evidence' is often used. This gives the user a convenient escape clause with which to cast doubt on the studies that have found effects, and to imply that a 'null-effect finding' means that radiation emitting technologies must be safe. However when a study finds no evidence of risk it doesn't mean that the technology is safe and we can use it without risk – rather it means that in using a particular study designed in a particular set of conditions, scientists didn't observe any effects. As we discussed earlier in this chapter, changing any of the parameters of the study may have changed the outcome.

McLean makes the point that no matter where you live or what you do, it's likely that you're in close contact with EMR-emitting technology for much of your day. If you have a cordless phone, sleep on an electric blanket, or use a mobile phone as an alarm clock, you're exposed as you sleep. If you use a computer, a mobile phone or electronic equipment in your job, you're exposed as you work. If you catch a bus, a train, or drive to work or occasionally catch a plane, then you're exposed as you travel.

McLean provides very good suggestions for reducing EMR at work and at home. Firstly, electric fields drop dramatically the further you move the equipment away from your body. If you have to have a computer on your desk, don't have it right in front of you when you work.

Wired connections appear to be less toxic than the wireless connection, so if you can use a landline rather than a mobile phone, do so. It is also possible to install some form of shielding from high-frequency signals both from an outside source and within the house.

One of the major sources of electromagnetic radiation is while we sleep. You're in your bedroom for up to eight hours per night and McLean gives the following tips:

1. Don't locate your bed on the other side of a wall from a source that produces high fields, such as a meter box, refrigerator or an off-peak hot water heater;

2. Try to keep all unnecessary electrical appliances, such as televisions or computers, out of the bedroom;

3. Make sure there are no electrical cables, power boards or copper pipes (which can emit fields) running under the bed. Try to keep the bed away from dimmer switches and ceiling fan control boxes;

4. Keep transformers and appliances, including digital clock radios, as far as possible from the bed. A battery operated clock has the lowest fields;

5. Don't use a mobile phone as an alarm clock and keep it out of the bedroom overnight while it is charging;

6. Don't sleep on an electric blanket overnight while it is turned on. If you use an electric blanket, warm the bed and then unplug the blanket at the power point before you get back into the bed;

7. You could consider installing a demand switch, which cuts power to a circuit when it is not being used, in order to remove all electrical fields from the bedroom as you sleep;

8. As an alternative to the demand switch, you could run a new power circuit to the bedroom with its own master switch. This too would allow mains power to be cut off to the bedroom at night without affecting appliances elsewhere in the house.

So, when you move to a new home or office, it would be wise to plan and design your new space. *The Force* also provides excellent suggestions on how to reduce electromagnetic radiation in all aspects of your life. Consider the design of the buildings, especially the wiring, placement of meter boxes and the conductive pipes used to insulate the wiring.

I can't leave the subject of electromagnetic radiation before considering the entire issue of diagnostic radiology. With the increasing use of CT scanning and nuclear medicine, many people are being exposed to excessive amounts of radiation on an acute basis. We tend to present the evidence based on the exposure to one chest x-ray, which is very low dose radiation. However, a typical intravenous CT angiogram, whether it be the brain, chest or gut, involves anywhere between 300 to 500 chest x-rays of radiation. A standard nuclear examination is around 300 chest x-rays of radiation. Again, this is very much related to the age at which you initially have these tests and the particular dose of radiation given, but suffice to say the younger you are and the more radiation you have, the greater chance that this radiation can induce a cancer.

When your doctor suggests any tests for any condition, always ask if there is an alternative test that does not involve radiation that gives the same information. In my specialty, cardiology, I am a great believer in stress imaging. There are two forms of stress imaging – stress echocardiography and stress nuclear. Both tests give relatively similar results but stress echocardiography (which I perform on a regular basis) does not involve radiation or injections, only takes around half an hour of your time and is basically an ultrasound of the heart before and after a full treadmill exercise test.

Nuclear cardiology involves an injection of nuclear material around 300 chest x-rays of radiation, is twice the price and can often take up to five hours to have performed.

I see this one as a real no brainer.

Synthetic chemical exposure

Now, just when you thought you'd solved the issue of environmental health by reducing your exposure to EMR, another major problem needs to be considered – synthetic chemical exposure!

Unfortunately, without even considering what you're doing to yourself, from the moment you wake up in the morning, you're being exposed to thousands of micro-doses of chemicals.

This comes back to the 'safe dose of poison' concept. The real answer here is we just don't know. If you believe 'industry', they'll reassure you that the levels of chemicals used in all aspects of our lives are so small that they should be considered harmless. The problem is that because there are so many chemicals used, we really can't tell what is a problem and what is not.

Industry may be right, but evidence is mounting from independent researchers that they're not. As I've mentioned, in the 1920s the cancer death rate was around 3 per cent. Part of the reason for this was that many people died earlier of infections, not living long enough to develop cancer.

But the cancer rates vary now between 30 and 35 per cent and are rising and cancer certainly occurs in young people as well, so I don't believe this increase in modern times is purely related to longevity. I think it is the intrusion into our environment of these varying poisons. This includes the synthetic chemicals used in our common household products, as well as the obvious pollution experienced in most major cities around the world. There is a clear link between air pollution and a variety of diseases, from lung conditions such as asthma to heart disease and cancer.

There are a number of independent environmental experts who have linked the variety of ubiquitous synthetic chemicals and numerous health problems. A number of studies suggest that conditions such as ADHD, autism, learning disabilities, diabetes, obesity, childhood and pubertal cancers, abnormal genitalia, infertility, breast and prostate cancers – not to mention a possible link between Parkinson's disease and Alzheimer's – have some link with these various chemicals.

An excellent summary of this entire issue is the book *Slow Death by Rubber Duck: How the Toxic Chemistry of Everyday Life Affects our Health* by Rick Smith and Bruce Lourie. These intrepid environmental researchers made the ultimate sacrifice by exposing themselves to a whole host of commonly used products which – it has been suggested – have created many of the above health issues. They then offered some solutions on how to detoxify the body. To quote from their book, 'The truth of the matter is that toxic chemicals are now found at low levels in countless applications, in everything from personal care products and cooking pots and pans to electronics, furniture, clothing, building materials and children's toys. They make their way into our bodies through our food, air and water. From the moment we get up from a good night's sleep under the wrinkle-resistant sheets (which are treated with the known carcinogen formaldehyde) to the time we go to bed after a snack of microwaved popcorn (the interior of the bag being coated with an indestructible chemical that builds up in our bodies), pollution surrounds us. Far from escaping it when we shut our front door at night, we've unwittingly welcomed these toxins into our homes in countless ways. In a particularly graphic example, it's been estimated that by the time the average woman grabs her morning coffee, she's applied 126 different chemicals and 12 different products to her face, body and hair.'

They presented evidence on the following chemicals:

Benzene: this is a toxic compound found in coal, common natural gas and crude oil. It is a key molecular building block for chemicals such as bisphenol A (BPA), phthalates, triclosan, PCBs and PBDEs, many of which are the serial offenders when evaluating environmental poisons.

The major source of mercury in our environment comes from coal-burning power plants. The human body is a sponge which soaks up these toxic chemicals. Not surprisingly the greatest sponge in the human body is fat. There is now good evidence to support the notion that the fatty apron around the abdomen is not just an ugly lump of lard, but also a toxic reservoir that holds on to all manner of synthetic chemicals and finds it hard to say goodbye to them.

One study of obese patients suggested that compared with those with the lowest levels of the common environmental poison BPA, those with the highest detected levels had 30 times the rate of diabetes and heart disease.

In *Slow Death by Rubber Duck*, when Smith and Lourie were exposed to a variety of foods, household products and other common objects, sprays and chemicals, they showed clearly significant levels of common known toxins.

Phthalates are the chemicals used to make vinyl soft and rubbery. A variety of phthalates are commonly used for different purposes. Children's toys are typical examples – thus the term 'slow death by rubber duck'. A typical rubber duck is around 37 per cent phthalates. Phthalates have been linked to a spectrum of developmental disorders involving the penis and testicles. It is a vital point that rapidly developing bodies, i.e. the embryo and young child, are even more sensitive to environmental toxins than adults.

Phthalates cross the placenta and are fat soluble, meaning they get stuck in that fatty reservoir that is your abdominal fat. Once there, it is hard to get out. Because they are fat soluble, they are not found in vegetables, but meat, dairy and processed foods have varying amounts of these toxic substances.

If you stop and do an inventory of your house, there is not much that hasn't been produced using phthalates. From everything plastic to cologne, aftershave, hair gel, deodorants and lotion, phthalates are there potentially causing their mischief.

Phthalates are part of the chemical spectrum of xeno-oestrogens. These are synthetic chemicals that mimic the effects of oestrogen in the body. The first human study of phthalates in health was performed in 2005, showing a highly significant relationship between maternal phthalate exposure during pregnancy and abnormalities in the penis and testicles of male offspring.

You may be shocked to find out that the Vinyl Council of Australia questioned the research methodology, emphatically stating that, to date, there is no clear evidence of harm to human beings from phthalate exposure, despite 50 years of use! (The research there is Swan S. H., 'Decrease in anogenital distance among male infants with prenatal phthalate exposure'. This comes from *Environmental Health Perspectives*, 2005; 113:1056-61.)

Closely linked to phthalates is BPA. The manufacturers give you a clue as to the BPA content by the RIC or Resin Identification Code. This is marked (typically on the bottom of a plastic container) in an arrowed triangle. The triangle is usually so small it's very hard to read the number without a microscope. RICs 1, 2, 4, 5 and 6 are very unlikely to contain significant amounts of BPA, whereas 3 and 7 are the typical suspects.

The BPA story appears even more frightening and far reaching than the phthalate issue. In 2007, a consensus statement was released by an expert panel suggesting the average BPA levels in humans were above those proven to cause harm in laboratory animals.

Apart from concerns about the foetus, there are links between BPA and obesity, diabetes and heart disease. Poor brain development has also been linked to BPA, with claims of links to autism and ADHD, along with heightened sensitivity to drugs of abuse.

There are also claims regarding BPA's links to a variety of cancers.

THE BREAST CANCER EPIDEMIC

The rates of breast cancer are on the rise. Breast cancer during pregnancy alone has doubled since the 1960s. A recent study published in *Obstetrics and Gynaecology* reviewed more than 4.1 million pregnancies in Sweden between 1963 and 2002. The incidence of cancer rose from 16 per 100,000 deliveries to 37 per 100,000 deliveries over this period, with the largest proportion being in the age group from 25 to 30.

However, we're not just talking about pregnancy related breast cancer, but breast cancer in general. The best current explanation for this rise in breast cancer gets back to one of the main themes of this book. Use the organ for what it is designed for, i.e. breastfeeding.

The female body is physiologically designed to commence menstruation somewhere after age 10 to 12. Soon after this, the female body was designed to get pregnant, breastfeed and nurture a child with a grandmother in her late 20s, early 30s assisting in the process.

This simple, top of the food chain job description certainly does not fit into our modern social framework. These days pregnancies are more typical in the late 20s with many women delaying childbirth to mid to late 30s and even early 40s. Socially this may seem reasonable but it's certainly disconnecting the woman from her true nature and physiology.

The breasts, which are very hormone-sensitive organs, often cop the brunt of this lifestyle choice. I'm not making any moral or ethical judgements, purely a medical observation. As I've mentioned, physiologically, the female body does its best work in the entire process by becoming pregnant in the 15- to 25-year age group.

The eggs are young and fresh, and the sperm is young and fresh. Let's face facts, 30-year-plus DNA in eggs and sperm is starting to change (as per my argument all through this book). After puberty, the breasts wait every month for the signals from the body to start gearing for a pregnancy and then the job of breastfeeding.

When this doesn't happen, the anticipating breasts retreat back to their established non-lactating status, hoping that the next month they can commence their pre-employment training. And so, month in, month out, the disappointment of not fulfilling their job description continues.

For many years we've been well aware of the link between breast cancer and the time of the first pregnancy. The longer the time, the greater the risk. So, by having this delay, women are living against their physiology and creating this risk.

But this is not the only factor involved here. A second major factor is what women are using to delay their pregnancies. Here I'm referring to synthetic hormones, i.e. the oral contraceptive pill that flogs the breast with pharmacological doses of oestrogen and progesterone in varying levels for a number of years.

The third and very pervasive factor here is, in fact, the xeno-oestrogens. Phthalates, BPA and other synthetic oestrogen mimickers bombard the female endocrine systems, breasts and ovaries from a very early age. High levels during pregnancy (as mentioned earlier), along with using hard plastic bottles, which are constantly rewarmed, to feed young children, leech these toxins into the milk.

This is a highly plausible argument as to why young girls are commencing menstruation earlier and earlier. So oral contraceptives have the effect of not only flogging the breast with hormones, but also increasing the time from the onset of menstruation to the first pregnancy.

Thus, with all of the above, I think you can clearly see the argument as to why breast cancer rates are rising dramatically.

Smith and Lourie in *Slow Death by Rubber Duck* present further arguments as to the variety of other common toxins so ubiquitous in our modern everyday life. Teflon, which revolutionised non-stick cooking, has been associated with birth defects, hormone disruption, developmental problems and even an increase in cholesterol.

Cooking fumes when Teflon cookware is unattended and overheated may lead to serious lung damage. To quote from page 90, 'Dish detergent is a mild (in fact, more than just mild) proxy for many of the chemical exposures we face today. We are eating, drinking and soaking in tens of thousands of potentially toxic substances, most of which we know little about. When all of these chemicals are combined together in our drinking water, we know virtually nothing about how they interact with each other or our bodies, and we know particularly little about how they affect developing brains and foetuses. Medical experts have no idea whether 20 different carcinogenic chemicals in the water are 20 times more likely to cause cancer or 100 times or whether their effect is likely to be no different than that of just one chemical. In fact, this area of study, called cumulative risk assessment, is still in its infancy, and studies of the health effects of multiple chemical exposures are rarely undertaken due to the complexity and lack of scientific understanding of chemical interactions in humans. It is hard enough to understand the effects of one chemical, because it often takes 50 to 100 years of use and study to figure that out.'

Brominated flame retardants, used to 'fireproof' many substances, including children's pyjamas, appear to upset the immune system and also cause the typical problem of developmental abnormalities. Bruce Lourie, an enthusiastic fish consumer, decided to markedly increase his intake of fatty fish, and his blood levels of mercury tripled after seven meals. Mercury was also commonly used in dental amalgam, not to mention being a common base in many vaccines. Mercury has been associated with the following health consequences: in high doses it can cause permanent brain damage, other central nervous system disorders, memory loss, heart disease, kidney failure, liver disease, cancer, sensory problems and tremors. Apart from that, it's perfectly safe!

Over the past 50 years we've seen a progressive move from outdoor entertainment (especially for children) to what was cleverly described by the naturopath David Stelfox – during an interview on my radio show – as a two-dimensional life. Many people, including children, are now receiving their entertainment from a flat screen. I won't go into the behavioural problems I see from this, and I've already alluded to the electromagnetic radiation from this exposure, but the other issue is the sterility.

This brings up the entire problem of our increasingly sterile world.

BUGS VERSUS HUMANS

Over the centuries we've witnessed an ongoing battle between humans and all manner of microbes. From the great plague to syphilis, the Spanish flu to tuberculosis and malaria, humans have been devastated by a variety of these tiny bugs.

Until the antibiotic era beginning in the 1940s, we really had not much to offer in defence. Since the advent of stronger and stronger antibiotics, we've seen many bacterial illnesses conquered, only to see resistant strains emerging.

Unfortunately, now many bacteria are emerging that are resistant to all current available antibiotics. Many infectious disease experts are predicting that over the next 10 years our current antibiotics will be virtually useless. Many authorities blame the increasing resistance on the excessive use of antibiotics, but others blame factors that I'll detail over the next few paragraphs. Over the past decade, we've seen the emergence of bird flu and then swine flu as viruses figure out clever ways to become more virulent.

Also, no-one could forget the emergence of HIV-AIDS. The epidemic officially began in June 1981, although retrospective analysis takes the first human case back to the 1950s.

It isn't just antibiotics and newer brands of antivirals that are being blamed for these resistant strains, but also many of the common household products we use, such as antibacterial wipes/cleansers/mouthwash and disinfectants. Although many authorities are strong advocates for (especially) alcohol-based antiseptics, we are recognising the health issues arising as a consequence of those products containing triclosan.

It is felt that triclosan-based products: 1. have no better action than products that do not contain triclosan; 2. are linked to health issues; 3. also contribute to bacterial resistance and super-bugs. Triclosan is linked to thyroid cancers in some laboratory animals and is also an offender in the abnormal hormonal effects seen with other toxins, although this appears to have more effect on the male rather than female hormonal system.

Maybe using triclosan and BPA may balance your hormones! I think not.

Firstly, let me make the point that triclosan is found in many household products below the level of 0.3 per cent, and is therefore deemed (by the companies that produce these products through their 'independent' testing) to be safe.

Just to name a few products where you'd expect to find triclosan: toothpaste, antibacterial soaps, foaming facial cleanser, shaving gel, deodorant and dishwashing liquid. Even the toxicity of triclosan aside, the attempt to shelter children from natural environments and keep them in our increasingly fortress-like homes (away from harm's way) decreases their exposure to the important natural bacteria found in dirt and has been shown to block the allergic response.

Whatever the reason, we have seen at least a doubling of food allergies, asthma and eczema in children over the past 20 years and the oversterilisation of our environment seems to be a culprit.

Then there is the old chestnut of the antibiotics and hormones used to bulk up a variety of meat products. To quote an excellent article by John van Tiggelen in the *Sydney Morning Herald*, in 2008 a survey was commissioned by the $8 billion beef industry which stated that one in three consumers would never touch Australian beef if they were told that hormones had been used in its production. The problem is that about half of Australia's 28 million beef cattle are at some point plugged with hormones to produce our sausages, steaks, burgers, roast, and the mince for our spaghetti bolognese. The conclusion of the study was that 'there is a significant risk to consumer confidence from a rise in consciousness'. The problem is that the hormone implants, which are of course marketed by our old friends the pharmaceutical industry, boost the growth in cattle by up to around 30 per cent. A four dollar cartridge of hormone behind the ear of a cow lasts for around three months and this typically returns at least 10 times the value in extra meat, with the need for less feeding and time saved (the cow grows quicker and can be slaughtered earlier).

The industry cleverly disguises the hormones by using the term HGPs, which stands for Hormone Growth Promotants. These are typically the different variety of sex hormones which may have a significant effect in disrupting the body's hormonal balance.

Interestingly, people tend to think most of the hormones are in chicken, but in fact hormones are not used in chicken.

So, I've tried to present a brief overview of the potential subtle and not so subtle exposures we experience in our day-to-day lives from a variety of sources of electromagnetic radiation and synthetic chemicals.

The reality is we all choose to live in society and many of these potential toxins are unavoidable to some extent, but we don't have to go out of our way to bathe our bodies in this stuff!

CHAPTER 14

Stage 3 – genetic health (the gene(ie) is out of the bottle)

The six basic life questions – who, what, where, why, when and how – are what makes up the you of now. This you today is the sum total of every life experience and memory you have had since you were conceived. But the other major factor here is what created you in the first place. This creation is a set of chemicals known as nucleotides, which make up the three billion base pairs in each molecule of your DNA.

This DNA not only determines the obvious aspects of your body such as your external appearance and the position and size of your organs, but also how this functioning unit called 'you' responds to everything that occurs in your life.

The system is truly magical because the DNA creates a you that is bigger than the DNA itself. Although the DNA is crammed into a part of the cell called the nucleus, it creates through a series of chemical messages all other components throughout the cell, including all of the receptor sites on the cell membrane and the effector proteins that arise as a consequence of the variety of stimuli reaching your external environment to these receptors.

Now here's a vital point. Every life experience (and as we know, these can be close to infinite) is recorded in your cells. This wonderfully intelligent system not only records the memory, but also adjusts accordingly to accommodate this memory. The other extraordinary fact here is that although your cells turn over at a constant rate, to ensure that once a finite individual cell has performed its necessary function but (as all life does) is wearing out and becoming defective, it experiences a process known as apoptosis, which is better described as programmed cell death.

The lining of the gut is being constantly bombarded with raw material (known as food), plus, unfortunately, a whole host of other substances (typically legal, but at times illegal), for which it has to respond with a multitude of chemicals. From high-potency acid in the stomach, to the bile from the gall bladder and the protein-splitting enzymes in the pancreas, these poor living cells don't get much of a rest. You may only eat three meals per day, but it takes your gut hours to digest, absorb and appropriately distribute all of this food and other stuff you dump in it.

Thus, after four to five days of this very hard work, the gut lining is exhausted, the cells die and slough off into the gut lumen (or channel) and, like the food and other stuff hanging around, has to be digested, absorbed and distributed by the viable cells.

The new cells don't get a few days' supervised training, they are already primed and have to start working as efficiently as the ones they replaced.

So, let's say that you're 45 years old and when you were 22 you had your usual 'rite of passage' trip to Phuket. After that dodgy curry in the beachside café, instead of lazing by the pool in your three-star resort, you spent a few days in your room on the bed and in the bathroom, finding inventive ways to empty your gastrointestinal tract from both ends. The bug that enjoyed its time in your gastrointestinal tract was possibly one of the many strains of *E. coli*.

After making it back home, for the next few months your bowels were loose and you felt pretty damn tired but eventually recovered, with no fond memories of Phuket and its surrounds.

Now, as a successful and moderately wealthy 45 year old, you decide to dip your toe once again in the crystal clear waters of Phuket. You take your wife and young family, this time to a five-star resort, with a much better restaurant, bar, a huge pool and – thankfully – more salubrious bathroom facilities.

But your old mate *E. coli* has missed you over the years. Let's face it, you shared some rather intimate moments with him or her 23 years ago and it has been hankering for your return. This very distant memory, both in your mind and gut, has basically been left behind as you take the family to the traditional Thai on the beach at Phuket.

Your wife loves curry and your children tuck in to the satays. You join your family in this appetising meal in this Thai paradise, unaware that your old mate *E. coli* has been tracking you since your arrival, just waiting for the chance.

Lying in wait on a dodgy piece of lettuce, the *E. coli* gleefully takes the ride down your oesophagus, jumps head first into the steaming acidy waters of your stomach, looking forward to setting up shop for another few days of merriment in your small intestine. But just as the *E. coli* starts to fornicate in the folds of your duodenum, without any prompting from your conscious mind, out come the big guns. Before you know it, your army – also known as your immune system – has received messages from the sentries on duty throughout your gastro-intestinal tract that the nasty little critter, *E. coli*, has attempted re-entry, but this time, your immune system is ready for it.

Somewhere, somehow, 23 years later, well over a thousand new gastrointestinal tracts later (do the maths on a new gastrointestinal lining every five days), that unpleasant memory of the *E. coli* assault on your gut has not been forgotten.

Within minutes to hours, every last bit of this nasty bug has been chewed up and spat out by a series of cellular and chemical reactions, unbeknowns to you while you were enjoying the beach vista and sipping a post-dinner refreshment with your wife, with the children fast asleep.

Not even a whimper from your gut as you enjoyed the rest of the holiday! So what's happened? What's happened is that every life experience, every moment, creates a memory (good or bad). Why do some songs make you cry, smile, want to throw the radio or CD out the window, while others have no effect whatsoever?

It's the same stuff in a different guise. One of the reasons the vast majority of people find it hard to break old habits is that the reason for these habits and the circumstances you create around them are so engrained that your cell memory keeps them occurring in your life. But as we've gone past that magical use-by date of age 40, the system doesn't always work as efficiently.

Something as dramatic as a severe *E. coli* infection in your 20s will still probably be engrained in your cellular immune memory in your 40s, but that whooping cough vaccination as an infant and teenager may not prevent you developing whooping cough in your 60s, and certainly won't stop you passing this on to your newborn grandchild, especially if the mother of your grandchild wasn't vaccinated.

But it is precisely these life experiences, cell memories and the way our DNA and the intricate system of cellular behaviour, receptors, affector chemicals and messengers react to all of the above that determines the day to day, as well as decade to decade, quality of your life, health and risk of disease. Human beings are often searching for reasons why things have gone wrong. Why can't I find love? Why don't I get on with my co-workers? Why aren't I tall enough, smart enough, good looking enough? Why have I developed heart disease, cancer etc, etc?

Well, your answer is in one of the above. But where you are now is where you are. You can't go back on the six questions of you, but as Albert Einstein once said, 'You can't solve your current problems with the same thinking you used to create them.'

To change what's happening now, all you can alter is the environment you're subjecting yourself to at the present time.

Regret about your body's characteristics, mistakes you made in the past, life's traumas (that occur to everyone, by the way, so don't feel singled out) and any other good or bad piece of misfortune that has occurred in the past is just that – PAST.

You can start to work, from today onwards, getting it right. Rewriting the script. You can't change your cellular memory but you can change your cellular behaviour, by changing all of the stuff that you subject yourself to on a day-to-day basis.

I'm not just talking here about the obvious physical stuff. I'm also talking about the environment of your thoughts and feelings. Thoughts and feelings don't just occur in your brain. They occur in every cell in your body. The DNA in your brain cells is the same stuff in your big toe. Every cell is you and every cell responds to the environment in which you decide to exist.

Even your thoughts and feelings are to some extent primed by these cellular memories. How often do you take an instant dislike to someone? The reason for this almost certainly stems from cellular memory. That person triggers a series of chemical reactions in your body based on a memory from before.

It may be an uncle you didn't like or the school bully, an old lover etc: the point is you've just met this new person and for a reason you can't exactly bring to your conscious mind, they irritate the life out of you.

One of the other important points here is that it is not just your own life experiences that determine this – your DNA is a compilation of your parents, their parents, their parents' parents, all the way back to good old Adam and Eve, or whatever biblical or evolutionary story you'd like to stake your genetic claim to. And given that DNA creates your cells, it also (to some extent) creates your cellular reaction to all these events, including that really irritating person who hasn't had the decency to leave the room.

But, to an extent, everything can be reprogrammed. I'm not suggesting that we can reprogram parts of our bodies to grow taller or lengthen (sorry, gentlemen, I'm not a magician) – some things are set in stone!

I'm also not suggesting a 50 year old can reprogram their thoughts and feelings to have them back looking like a 30 year old. Even plastic surgeons can't do that. You can, however, reprogram your thoughts and feelings, your eating habits, your exercise habits, your addictive habits and therefore, overall, your entire behavioural patterns, which will give you the best chance of feeling younger, looking better, being healthier and living longer.

Many of our common diseases, such as heart disease and cancer, have a genetic basis. But often, unless there are specific environmental triggers, the genes may lie dormant and the person remains well throughout their life. (Well, this is probably an exaggeration, because we all have to die of something and I suspect we won't be particularly well at the time.)

To give one cancer example, around 20 per cent of the smoking population will develop lung cancer, whereas 80 per cent will not. Every day you smoke you induce around 15 to 20 mutations in your lungs and when you've reached a critical mass of around 20,000 mutations, these combine to form a malignant tumour. But if you're a non-smoker, it's unlikely these genetic mutations will occur – thus the low (but not zero) rate of lung cancer in non-smokers.

It is also important to know that there are a variety of lung cancers, the less common types being unrelated to cigarette smoking.

I have often heard comments such as, 'My grandmother never smoked and she died of lung cancer.' What people don't say is that poor old Grandma was married to Grandpa who was a heavy smoker, so second-hand smoke was a major contributor.

'My grandfather smoked till he was 85 and he was knocked over by a bus.' This probably occurred because he was trying to light a cigarette while he was crossing the road and failed to see the bus. I feel sorry for bus drivers and buses. They get blamed for a hell of a lot of accidents.

Phil's story

Phil was my best friend from childhood and worked for a major Australian airline for a number of years, before the days of significant occupation health and safety. He was an aircraft engineer who climbed into the fuel tanks to repair them. He'd sit inside the tanks and when he started to feel close to unconsciousness, he'd get out. Of course, for a number of years he used to breathe in quite noxious fumes.

He stopped working for the airline around 15 years before he developed a cough. The respiratory physician who saw him initially thought he may have an exotic infection such as tuberculosis.

Despite a few months of treatment Phil's cough wasn't improving. After further tests it was found that he had a condition known as bronchiolar-alveolar cell cancer, which is a non-cigarette-related lung cancer. In Phil's case it was pretty obvious that this was directly connected to toxic exposure, and in fact he received compensation from the airline. Unfortunately, he died a tragic death a few years later. Phil detested cigarette smoking and it was somewhat ironic that he died of a condition that is typically associated with smoking, although in his case his particular type of lung cancer had no relationship whatsoever to cigarette smoke.

Genetic heart risk

When you hear about a (typically) male in his 40s who has never smoked, has normal blood pressure and cholesterol but drops dead jogging, he usually has an elevated level of a purely genetic cholesterol-carrying protein known as lipoprotein(a), which I mentioned earlier in the book. One in five people have this genetic abnormality and if it is present in elevated amounts (above 0.3 grams per decilitre) their risk for a cardiovascular event such as a heart attack is 70 per cent higher than someone without this genetic abnormality.

The only way that you know you have lipoprotein(a) running around in your bloodstream in excessive amounts is to have the blood test.

However, most doctors don't measure it because they say there is nothing you can do about it, so why bother! The reality is that there are good reasons to know whether your lipoprotein(a) is elevated:

1. There are now a multitude of studies showing that if your Lp(a) is abnormal, you are at high risk for a cardiovascular event. Thus, if you know you have this abnormality, it should (a) make you even more diligent about lifestyle modification, and (b) prompt you to have a full cardiovascular work-up;
2. It is my strong opinion from treating thousands of patients with this abnormality that the use of nicotinic acid with specific vitamins can reduce Lp(a) levels and also minimise the effects of Lp(a) on your blood vessels.

Thus I use a combination of vitamin C dose 1 gram twice daily, the natural version of vitamin E (d-alpha tocopherol, not the synthetic version dl-alpha tocopherol), in a dose of 500 international units taken in the evening with the second dose of vitamin C, along with L-lysine 500 milligrams in the morning. Professor Pauling and Dr Rath suggest a much higher dose of these supplements, but I've had great success over the years using this combination along with nicotinic acid. I only use nicotinic acid if someone already has established heart disease or has a high calcium score placing them in the 25th percentile for their age.

Lp(a) aside, a number of studies have confirmed the presence of 25 different genetic abnormalities increasing heart disease risk independent of cholesterol and blood pressure, emphasising that these are not the only contributing factors to our commonest killer.

Regardless of the disease, there are specific tests to determine either the genetic abnormality or the effect on the body of that specific abnormality. This section is certainly not meant to be an exhaustive review of genetics but purely to point out that we are currently in a good position to assess many common conditions and determine to an important degree the contribution of genetics to the overall issue.

At present, we can't change your genes (for the most part), but we can alter the manner in which your genes interact with the environment and thus affect the natural history of your underlying condition.

Genetic screening

With the mapping in 2003 of the human genome – the entire sequence of human DNA – and the continuing work and refinements since, a number of commercial companies are already offering genetic screening procedures for a number of our common diseases.

At some point in the not too distant future, it may be standard medical practice to take DNA from (for example) human saliva and form a predictive map of each individual's lifetime risk for disease. Strategies in potential genetic engineering would then be possible to prevent that disease from ever occurring.

There are, however, a number of downsides to this approach:

1. Fear – if, for example, you were told that your risk for aggressive breast cancer was over 80 per cent, you'd live your life with a sword hanging over your head. Some people would prefer not to know and take their chances. When people attending my clinic for preventative cardiac screening receive results they don't expect, they can be devastated. Screening is always a difficult issue, because in many ways you're damned if you do and you're damned if you don't.

2. Employment – if the information falls into the wrong hands, it certainly may have an adverse effect on future employment. Employers may not wish to invest time, money and training on employees at high risk for various diseases.

3. Insurance – as screening tests become more and more accurate, if these (and in particular genetic screening) become the norm, it will be more difficult for some people to sign up for life insurance, as well as health and disability insurance. Once these tests become established, this may have serious implications at many levels of society.

The executive stress test

I believe that our current insurance screening methods are antiquated and have little predictive value in people not already displaying symptoms of a condition. This includes the executive stress test, which has long been a major component test for larger insurance policies.

As a cardiologist, it's my opinion that a stress test alone (i.e. without some form of imaging, either echo or nuclear) has little value because of its very high false positive and false negative rate. This is especially so in women. Because of the high radiation levels seen with stress nuclear tests, I almost exclusively perform stress echoes as a means of stress testing.

HIV

Around 1 per cent of Caucasians have a natural immunity to HIV. HIV was previously a lethal diagnosis but over the past 10 to 15 years, antiretroviral drugs have been developed to convert HIV into a chronic, manageable illness. These treatments cost around $25,000 per person per year to administer, but are well worth it to prevent the carnage resulting from such a miserable disease. Unfortunately, the antiretroviral drugs are not as widely available in places like Africa where the disease is still wreaking havoc.

Around four years ago, an AIDS patient appeared to be cured after getting donor blood cells from a man with this natural immunity to HIV. The way HIV wields its mischief is to enter the immune cells known as T-cells. These T-cells are vital to fight opportunistic infection. HIV enters these cells through a docking station known as a receptor. The docking station on the T-cell is called CCR5 (why don't they ever call these things names like Toby or Bill?).

People with natural immunity to HIV lack the CCR5 docking station on the surface of their T-cells. Thus the virus can't get in at all and therefore no HIV-AIDS for that person.

Sangamo BioSciences, a creative biotech company in California, was able to cut DNA at certain locations and edit out a gene. A team of researchers from the University of California in San Francisco conducted a trial of this therapy in six men with HIV. They removed a small percentage of their T-cells and in the laboratory removed the CCR5 gene with their stripping compound.

There are a group of chemicals called growth factors. These were added to the genetically modified T-cells bumping up the numbers to somewhere between two to five billion cells. In all six men, the anti-HIV cells were still doing their stuff 12 months post-infusion and the men have remained HIV-free. It's still too early to suggest a total cure, but it is certainly a major breakthrough in the management of HIV with significant implications for other diseases.

Almost all diseases have a genetic basis. The techniques used here have the potential to be developed for all the complaints affecting humankind, from Alzheimer's disease to the animal-acquired diseases, the zoonoses, i.e. the A to Z of diseases.

CHAPTER 15

Stage 4 – emotional health

'There is no more certain sign of insanity than to do the same thing over and over again and expect a different result,' said Albert Einstein. You can't stand your partner, your children are off the rails. You hate your job. You decide to have a heart attack in the middle of all this and then go back to the situation. Nothing is going to change.

You have two choices. Change your situation or change your attitude to your situation. It's actually quite straightforward, but it's not as easy as it sounds.

1. YOU

    You are the sum total of all your life experiences, along with your inherited DNA, up to this point. One disconcerting fact is that only 5 per cent of your reactions and behaviour are conscious, while 95 per cent is subconscious, and typically the script was written when you were very young.

    Your conscious mind can wander all over the place. You can drift back to a pleasurable incident 10 years previously or that delicious meal you enjoyed yesterday or that exciting event you're looking forward to next week.

It can also mull over all the traumas and bad luck you've encountered up to this point and all the potential issues that may arise over the next week, month, year or even decade (if you are that much of a pessimist). Your subconscious, however, is firmly stuck in the present, dealing with your immediate situation and reacting based on the scripts that were written years before. This also includes years before you were born. I've already stressed the importance of our basic instinct for survival. The tactics we use to ensure this survival certainly differ between individuals and can also vary within the individual depending on the threat.

As I mentioned previously, when we were living as hunter-gatherers and there was the threat of attack, our body immediately flipped into defensive mode. Our fear-flight system or our stress system rapidly jumped into action to allow us to have greater blood flow to our muscles and strength of heart contraction so we could defend ourselves with extra strength or run. We've retained these survival mechanisms, although they are slightly different in each of us – we certainly have no control over them.

The subconscious rapidly jumps into action based on the experiences we have had to date. Thus, some people thrive on conflict, danger and confrontation, while others will run at the first sign of trouble. We learn these traits as a child and one of the major skills of healing and health is to unlearn the traits that don't serve you.

So, as I'll stress in the next chapter, if you see your situational traumas from a totally different perspective, this is the first step to emotional health. Rather than adopt the defeatist, 'poor me' stance, my strong advice is to nurture your observer to create enormous awareness. If you cultivate this silent, non-judgemental observer who basically acts as a monitor of your behaviour, you then have an internal guide who can help you through many situations. With this awareness, see your life from a symbolic viewpoint. Ask, 'Why am I in this position? What am I supposed to learn as a consequence of this life event?' Yes, event, not trauma.

If you see that the universal energy that you attract creates these situations for you to learn from, then your attitude towards your life has to change. You are the central character in your life drama and it is up to you to play the role properly and in the best manner that serves you and the key people in your life.

If there's a problem in your life, it is vital you don't immediately blame those involved rather than asking what you are doing to attract this issue. Your ingrained subconscious script will always attempt to justify your position as the correct one. For example, I've never met anyone who has told me that the failure of a business partnership was their fault.

Speak to anyone who has divorced. It was always the other person who caused the marriage breakup, not them. I have no doubt that in any defective relationship, be it personal or business, there are two or more people involved, all bringing their own problems and issues to the table.

The reality is that the only person you can truly influence in this situation is you. I am in no way suggesting you should become other people's punching bag. What I'm saying is that if you ask 'How may I serve?' and 'What is this situation teaching me in my development as a better and healthy individual?' I can assure you, your life will change.

So, what situations can you expect throughout your life to cause you the most stress and, unfortunately, possibly contribute to serious illness? There are a variety of analyses of the issue of 'Top Life Stressors'. There is, however, basic agreement on our major life stresses and the severity of their impact on our lives. The Working Resources website has offered a typical breakdown, with a score for how much impact each stress imparts, 100 being the worst:

1. Death of a spouse – 100;
2. Divorce – 73;
3. Marital separation – 65;
4. Detention in jail or other institutions – 63;
5. Death of a close family member – 63;
6. Major personal injury or illness – 53;
7. Marriage – 50;
8. Losing your job – 47;
9. Marital reconciliation – 45;
10. Retirement from work – 45;
11. Change in health of a family member – 44;
12. Pregnancy – 40;
13. Sexual difficulties – 39;

14. Gaining a new family member – 39;

15. Major business readjustment – 39.

When you look down this list, it is rather difficult to escape many of these events. I'd venture to say that most of us will experience at least five and up to 10 of these events at some stage in our lives. I'm not entirely sure how they derive the actual scoring ranking, but the effect of the event does seem rather consistent with the number.

But this is where the new way of thinking comes in. See your world symbolically, ask why and what you can learn from this event, and your ability to cope and heal will improve markedly.

Many of the above events involve relationships, and a key point when discussing any relationship issue is that it is your responsibility to make you happy. This simple, but powerful statement can change the way you perceive all your relationships, whether they be at work or in your emotional life.

In any situation, try to be kind rather than right. The first and most important relationship here is the relationship you have with yourself. If you feel worthwhile and lovable you will be worthwhile and lovable to others. Be kind to yourself. Don't use negative language in your internal and external thoughts. Again, your subconscious script may tell you otherwise, but with ongoing awareness and training, you can rewrite the script.

2. COMMUNICATION

We've been told for years the vital importance of cultivating high-quality communication. This should occur in all areas of your life. Communicate your thoughts, your feelings and your needs in a positive, caring fashion.

Some tips for high-level communication are:

1. Criticise the behaviour, not the person – saying 'What you did was very upsetting and hurtful' is much more palatable and effective than comments like 'You're a horrible person, a fool, a pig' etc, etc. You're much more likely to resolve an issue with this attitude than by attacking the person directly.

2. In your relationship with your primary partner, don't go to bed angry. Resolve any issue you may have before sleep, because your sleep will be disturbed if you don't. Also and more importantly, it is bad energy to prolong fights and disagreements. Resolve them as soon as the acute anger settles.

3. On a positive note, a good hint is to practise the odd ET principle. Phoning home, especially on the way home from work, re-establishes the connection between you and your partner and also symbolically says that work has finished for the day. This gets your head out of the 'workspace' and into the home space. By the way, do you know what ET is short for? He's got little legs!

4. Don't lose the importance of your primary relationship because of your children. Often a couple purely becomes Mum and Dad. They even start calling each other that. Particularly when your children are young and physically very demanding, it is important for you to have time

together, at least weekly. Go to a movie, go out to dinner, and if you have long-suffering grandparents, have the occasional weekend away.

5. Show appreciation – this tip isn't just for your primary partner. Show appreciation to all those people in your life with whom you interact. Recognising and appreciating even the smallest acts of kindness and generosity shown to you by others should never go unnoticed. Again this highlights the importance of your observer never taking any acts of kindness and generosity directed towards you for granted.

3. FORGIVENESS

There is a wonderful Buddhist saying, 'If you want revenge on anyone, dig two graves.' Carrying around resentment and antagonism towards someone whom you perceive has harmed you can eat away at you.

Regardless of the severity of the trauma, your ability to forgive is the most healing act for you and is a vital aspect of emotional health. Think now of all the people throughout your life who have created problems for you. Visualise that person, send them love and forgive them. Make this forgiveness part of your meditative practice until any residual antagonism has melted away.

4. VALUE OTHERS

If you cultivate the service mentality and don't see other people as your servants, I can assure you your situation will start to heal. How often are you at a restaurant and the waiter – who happens to be a fellow human being – is leaning over you to pick up your plate. Does it really hurt for you to pick the plate up yourself, look the waiter in the eye and say thank you?

Ken's story

I believe the universe gives you examples when you need them. I once saw a woman in her 70s, named Val, with very high blood pressure. She was carrying on excessively about the fact that I'd suggested she needed a blood pressure pill. Val said, 'I heard you were the natural cardiologist – you should be able to organise some natural therapy to lower my blood pressure. I don't want to take pills.' This diatribe went on for a few minutes, but eventually I convinced Val that she needed medications, otherwise she'd pop a hole in her head as her blood pressure was far too high.

Interestingly, sitting in the waiting room was this delightful man by the name of Ken. Ken was also in his 70s and had undergone coronary artery bypass grafting, which in itself was a very big deal. But this was the least of Ken's concerns as he had a condition known as muscular dystrophy, where his muscles didn't work properly. Again this was probably the least of Ken's concerns as he was clinically blind and used to have to catch two buses and a train for his appointments with me.

What I wanted to do, but didn't, was bring Ken into the room and introduce him to Val. Ken has every reason on this planet to complain but chooses not to – he seems to count his blessings and basically thanks you for breathing in the same room that he is in.

I wanted to say to Val, 'You have no reason to complain but continually do so – figure it out.' This is a simple but powerful message. Ken catches the bus into the city every morning and helps some priests serve mass at one of the local Catholic churches. I asked him why he did this and he said, 'Doctor, I feel I have to contribute.' Ken has such a beautiful spirit despite his rather difficult and very inconvenient life, but wouldn't dream of complaining and constantly thanks everyone with whom he has any interaction. I believe there is a lot we can all learn from Ken.

I think you can see from this chapter that I'm not talking about a major situational change, but rather a major attitudinal change. Whether it be your home, work or recreation environment, it is your attitude to any of these scenarios that will determine your healing. The more value you perceive in another person or situation, the more valuable that personal situation will become.

5. BEST FRIENDS

    See your primary partner, your spouse – the most important figure in your life – as your best friend. Many people tend to take their partner for granted, forgetting to show this major consideration.

    One of the most extraordinary experiences of my life came a few years ago when I was doing a road show for a major insurance company and I'd been away from home for around three days. I landed at Sydney Airport on a plane from Perth and then had to drive south of Sydney to give another lecture. I wasn't going to arrive back at my house, which is in the opposite direction, until a few hours later.

    When I arrived at the airport and switched on my mobile phone there was a message, 'ring Anne ASAP' (Anne being my beautiful wife). I rang her thinking there was something wrong, and I said, 'What's the problem, darling?' She said, 'Nothing – I'm at the airport.' I asked her why she'd come here. She replied, 'To have a cup of coffee with you.' I said, 'Why have you driven across Sydney in heavy traffic for a 20 minute cup of coffee when I'm going to be home in a few hours?' She said to me, 'I couldn't wait.'

After 30 years of marriage, this was one of the most extraordinary, simple acts I had ever experienced and I thought to myself what a privilege it was to be married to this person who obviously loves me as much as I love her.

When she arrived home, there was a big bunch of flowers waiting for her.

In a relationship between male and female, issues often arise because of the inherent differences between sexes. In his flagship book *Men Are from Mars, Women Are from Venus*, John Gray clearly details these differences. There are some clear ways in which the male brain is wired differently from the female brain. It's very important that these differences are recognised when weaving your way through the myriad issues that arise within your primary relationship.

Males are very much behaviour orientated. They judge themselves and others on behaviour – who is the best sportsman, the hardest worker etc, etc. Women, however, are more feeling orientated – on the whole, their emotional life is much more important to them.

The major motivation for a male is solving problems and

feeling needed for his ability to do so. The major motivation for the female is feeling loved and cherished, not because of her problem solving ability but purely because she is lovable.

The male tries to change or advise people (especially their partners) about their feelings, whereas the female purely wants to be heard and have her feelings validated. Males love giving advice because fixing things is what they're good at. It all comes back to biology – men are the hunters, the providers. It's their job to venture into the jungle, find and/or kill the food and bring it back to the cave to feed their family.

To hunt effectively requires a strategy and system and this is basically the male modus operandi. So, if there's a problem, it is important to have a system and strategy to solve it.

The female, however, is biologically primed to be the nurturer, the protector of the family and especially her children. Nurturing involves love and feelings, whereas solutions, strategies and systems are not so important to her. As long as she feels she is being listened to, then the female is happy. She doesn't necessarily want a solution.

When a man has a problem, he either wants to sweep the issue under the carpet (or back in the hunter-gatherer days when the carpets were in scarce supply – sand in the cave) or to brood on his own.

The female prefers to talk until the issue is resolved; a vital component of being a good nurturer. The female is a multi-tasker who has no problems dealing with a number of issues at the one time – for instance, preparing a meal and helping a child with their homework, while simultaneously discussing a problem with a friend on the phone. Her brain can switch from one task to another in a heartbeat, a vital skill for a nurturer.

The male, however, typically works in compartments, as he needs to 'focus on the kill'. One false move, one lapse in concentration, can see the male have his head ripped off by that sabre-tooth tiger or felled by a member of the opposing tribe.

These biological traits have continued into our modern world. If you don't believe me, try to interrupt a man while he's watching TV (especially sport). He is focused and there is nothing you can do about it. The house can be burning down, but if there's an important sporting match on you won't get his attention.

When he is at work, he is in the work compartment. When he is relaxing at home, that's the compartment he's in. If there's an argument at home, as soon as he goes off to work, the home compartment is shut and the argument is forgotten. With hours at work, the argument has been long forgotten and by the time he arrives home it is ancient history.

But, typically, this is not the case for the female, who needs to talk about the issue and resolve it, despite the fact that she has been multi-tasking her way through the day.

Of course, these are sweeping generalisations that don't apply to every member of either sex, but I think you can see my point. There are many reasons for situational dysfunction and they are usually around these points of difference between individuals.

I believe one of the greatest causes of emotional distress is either you, or those around you, behaving in a manner that is unreasonable. Whether this be excessive anger, unreasonable jealousy, any form of abuse, or mismanagement of personal finances – to name just a few examples – these unreasonable behaviours cause stress until they're resolved.

Emotional health is really a full book in itself but suffice to say that if you're unhappy with your current lot in life, for whatever reason, unhappiness and discontent can be significant factors in a majority of our major diseases and killers. In over 30 years of practising medicine, I have not seen too many patients with serious illnesses who didn't either have significant life stresses, social isolation, loneliness or general unhappiness lurking around at the time of their illness.

In the next chapter, I'll detail how these life stressors interact with our seven energy centres to determine what type of disease process typically befalls us. The comforting thought here is that with the right approach and process, you can change how these stresses impact on your life with a progression towards true health.

CHAPTER 16

Stage 5 – mind health

The premise of this chapter (and also of the book) is the concept of as is the microcosm, so is the macrocosm. Every cell in your body has an extraordinary intelligence that, under normal circumstances, determines when the cell divides, what nutrition it requires, what proteins it produces, how it rids itself of cellular waste, and even when it has outlived its usefulness and it's time to make way for a new breed of exactly the same cells.

All of this is programmed into the cellular intelligence. If you treat your body well at all levels, the cells do their job with the minimum of fuss and without complaint. But here's the issue. This next statement sets the scene for the rest of this chapter and this book. The essence of your existence is freewill, choice and quality decisions. The world is perfectly imperfect because this is the end game.

If the world was perfect, there would be no point. Nothing would ever go wrong, nothing would challenge us and (heaven forbid) there would be no need for doctors because we'd never get sick. Every living organism would live forever and this finite resource called the planet earth would become so over-crowded there would be no planet earth left. Thus the need for natural disasters, victors and victims, happiness and pain and the vital need for the life cycle, which includes death.

But another important feature is that just as our cells make up the functioning unit that is our body, our bodies are part of the functioning unit that is our planet. This is another key point. A major driver of our planet is evolution, and as any system evolves it becomes more complex. Human beings and all current life on earth has evolved from single cell organisms. I believe the functional purpose of our lives, beyond sheer survival, is to evolve. I especially believe this function is spiritual evolution – to become more conscious, aware, compassionate, loving people.

I'll now explain how I believe this system works and what we can all do to heal our own personal issues that have arisen as a consequence of the slow, but effective process of evolution. As I've stated throughout this book, energy is a key feature of good health, lack of disease and our ability to function normally on a day-to-day and year-to-year basis. But energy isn't purely a physical function. It also occurs at a mental, emotional and spiritual level.

I realise that, so far, this book has mainly dealt with the scientific aspects of health and that, as we delve into the area of healing the mind and the spirit, not everyone is going to agree with what I write in this chapter.

I do strongly believe that if you follow the seven universal spiritual laws that I'll outline shortly, health will follow. But for anyone who is sceptical about this type of thing, I'll try to explain it as well as I can, and hopefully you'll be able to connect with it in some way.

In Margaret Ruby's excellent book, *The DNA of Healing*, she states that our core beliefs are imprinted in our DNA. Typical defective life situations detailed in the previous chapter, such as abandonment, betrayal, loss of trust, separation and feelings of rejection have been imprinted in our DNA through ancestral experience.

These beliefs guide many of our emotions, thoughts and actions. 'Common memories of droughts, plagues, floods, famines, inquisitions, holocausts' and many phobias may be as a consequence of these inherited core experiences and beliefs. Each experience has interacted with our own unique DNA to create who we currently are. You can choose to accept this, along with all its possibilities of illnesses, life reactions and life quality, or – if you're not happy with your current situation – take steps to change.

The Seven Spiritual Laws

So, what are the seven spiritual laws and why do I believe they are so relevant to achieving health?

1. All is one
    This law basically connects us all. Every thought, emotion, action influences the system. I believe the universal spirit, which many people might refer to as God, is the highest vibrational energy. Atheists might perceive this energy as emanating from nature. We can either choose to live in this high vibrational zone or choose not to. But, suffice to say, I believe we're all connected. If you vibrate at a low energy (which I'll explain soon), you have an effect on the entire system, i.e. the planet.

    It takes only one cancer cell, one pathogenic virus, to start a serious illness. So don't assume that bad behaviour, bad choices, bad emotions have no consequence on anyone else.

1. Honour one another

    From your most cherished loved ones to the waiter or waitress in a restaurant, your relationships with other people have consequences. Respect all human life. Respect for all human life allows you to vibrate at this higher frequency. Cultivate your relationships. See every interaction as a test of who you are. Practise this every moment.

2. Honour yourself

    Many people lack self-esteem. Often this poor self-esteem is part of an ancestral 'chip on the shoulder'. If you believe you are not good enough, you won't be. It is difficult to love anyone else, if you can't love yourself.

3. Love is the ultimate power

    The ability to give and receive unconditional love is the strongest power in the universe. The God force is pure love at the highest vibrational level. A major feature of this law is forgiveness. Think about all the people through your life who have harmed you in any way. Forgiveness is the most healing technique for your cell tissue.

5. Surrender to the divine

    You could also say, surrender to life. This universal law directs you to live life at a totally different level. Beyond pure forgiveness for those who have harmed you is seeing the situations and opportunities they presented to you as your best teachers. If you see every occurrence in your life, whether it's small or large, with symbolic, spiritual lenses, life takes on a whole new meaning and purpose.

The divine – if I can use that term again – will give every living person a variety of good and bad experiences, but if you see each one as a learning and growth opportunity, then your life changes completely. No longer do you feel on a constant, irritating and stressful treadmill; you have now moved into a totally new realm of existence. Every accident, illness, life tragedy can be seen from this symbolic level. Surrender to life and from this you can make the best decisions that will serve you and those around you.

6. Seek the truth in all aspects of your life

So many of us live against our true nature. How many people are in work or relationships they don't value? How many people perform tasks for money, selling products they don't believe in? How often do you feel that sense of constant frustration with your life, feeling that something is missing?

So many of us have varying degrees of addiction, knowing full well that this is not what our bodies need. Once this universal law is violated, it leads to all manner of illnesses and to an extraordinary loss of wellbeing.

7. Live in the moment

So many people believe that the concept of heaven involves a place we 'travel' to once we pass on. The idea of a place in the clouds where we exist in eternal peace is the traditional concept of heaven. In many religions, this is also balanced by the punitive, typically subterranean place called hell, involving eternal damnation for those who have sinned.

There are, however, a number of people who don't believe in any existence after the one you may or may not be enjoying at this very moment (hopefully, if you're reading this book, you're closer to enjoyment than dissatisfaction).

Another plausible explanation is that, with the right tools, you can access heaven here on earth. This explanation involves being in touch with the spirit, the universal vibrational energy, that gives and directs our lives.

One strong method is to cultivate the silent observer which resides within us all. This observer can be accessed at any moment and allows us to be fully in the present. I believe this is our connection to God, or, if you like, to the highest vibrational level I mentioned earlier. The more we focus and are present in the moment, the greater the connection.

CHAKRAS

Three years ago, I was giving one of my corporate talks to an insurance group in Singapore. As I travel so often, it's a pleasure for me to take either my wife or one of my children with me to enjoy many of the exotic locations I've had the privilege of visiting. On this occasion, I took my eldest son, Paul. Anyone who knows Paul will tell you he has a fierce intellect and is never backward about offering his opinion.

He attended my lecture entitled 'Your biography becomes your biology' and afterwards my rather cynical, sceptical son said, 'Dad, that was a load of unproven rubbish. You took a bunch of examples and fitted them into your scheme.'

When you read this section, you may think the same, or conversely, it may induce one of those 'ah-hah' moments. It certainly didn't do that for my son!

The seven universal spiritual laws I've just mentioned coincide with the energy theory of the body. The ancient Hindus described a system of anatomic energy centres called chakras. These chakras have specific sites in the body.

A conscious or subconscious violation of one of these laws leads to an energy disruption in one of the chakras and a specific disorder related to this area of the body. In her book *Anatomy of the Spirit,* Caroline Myss provides a comprehensive explanation of this theory. One attraction to this way of thinking is that it provides the final level of health over and above the first four that I've already detailed.

C1

This is the base chakra. This connects you to the earth and your tribe – 'tribe' often means your family or society. If you feel disconnected from people around you, or the earth as a whole, you develop disorders of immunity, blood disorders or problems with your lower limbs.

HIV is a classic C1 disease. The gay community, prostitutes and IV drug users (not to mention Africa collectively as a continent) feel disconnected from the rest of the world. As the acceptance of homosexuality has – thankfully – increased, the devastation from HIV in this particular group has been reduced. In a modern society, HIV is now seen more as a chronic illness than a death sentence.

C2

This is the relationship chakra, located around your belly button. This is your centre of creativity – sex, money and power. Low back pain is typically associated with financial problems. Gynaecological issues are very much tied in with relationship issues.

Prostate cancer typically affects older males who lose their power base. For example, the CEO who retires and no longer feels worthwhile or useful often develops this condition.

C3

Solar plexus. This is the chakra of self-esteem. This is the area of personal power. People with self-esteem issues typically suffer gastrointestinal problems such as peptic ulcerations, reflux, dyspepsia and irritable bowel. This is also the area for diseases of the pancreas, liver and spleen.

C4

The heart chakra. Located in the centre of the chest, blocks in this area are indicated by heart disease, breast cancer and lung disease. This is based around your ability and opportunity to give and receive unconditional love.

Julie was in her early 40s. She'd had full breast cancer, and had to have both breasts removed. When she told me about her life prior to developing breast cancer, it was quite obvious to me why her fourth chakra had been violated. Her husband had left her and their four children to start a new relationship with an 18-year-old woman.

Julie's body couldn't handle this extraordinary violation of her fourth chakra, thus the breast cancer. The universe, however, works on energy. Not only did Julie suffer this significant disruption to her fourth chakra energy, her husband – who had committed a serious breach of his first chakra (he'd dislocated himself from his immediate tribe, his family) – died a few years later from leukaemia, a very prominent C1 illness.

Since then, Julie has healed from her disease. Why? Because she practised the most powerful form of C4 healing – forgiveness.

Natasha was in her 50s and came to see me because of minor heart palpitations. When taking her medical history, I discovered she had suffered breast cancer years before. On further questioning, until around three years ago she hadn't spoken with her mother for a 17-year period. Hardly a formula for a healthy fourth chakra.

Natasha eventually reconciled with her mother and has a more nurturing relationship now, which leads to a much healthier fourth chakra.

C5

The throat chakra – this is located around the area of speech, and is the chakra of choice and decision. Disruptions in this lead to problems with the throat, the larynx and the thyroid.

Philippa was in her late 20s. She had struggled with a variety of jobs, none of which captured her interests. Her emotional relationships seemed to follow the same pattern. She then met Richard, who was a property developer with very strong opinions. After a 12-month relationship, they were engaged. Philippa seemed to go along for the ride, but was never sure whether this was what she really needed or wanted.

She began to sweat profusely, experienced heart palpitations and felt anxious, with an increase in her bowel actions. At the same time she developed a large lump in her throat. She was diagnosed with an overactive thyroid with associated goitre.

Her fifth chakra was telling Philippa that her body was not happy with her decisions. At this point Richard was making most of them for her. Philippa saw an energetic healer and counsellor and when she confronted her issues, she realised that her life direction wasn't serving her. She broke off the engagement and pursued work in an area that she had an interest and passion for. The goitre was very large and pressing on the local structures in the neck so she had an operation, her symptoms abated, and she was able to stop the other medications for the thyroid. In this situation I believe the combination of good orthodox medicine and healing the fifth chakra issues were what saw Philippa on the road to recovery.

C6

This is located between the eyes. The mystics call this the third eye – the centre of truth and wisdom. Disruptions in this chakra are manifested by recurring headaches, stroke, epilepsy, brain tumours and other chronic cerebral conditions.

Migraines are typical C6 diseases. With a migraine you go to a darkened room, away from other people, take a painkiller until the headache settles and have some time away from reality for a while.

C7

This is known as the crown chakra. This is the direct connection to the divine. Energetically this is the site of divine inspiration. Diseases of this chakra are typically skin problems or auto-immune diseases with a strong musculoskeletal component.

As the corresponding universal law is to live in the moment, diseases in this area have a strong link to major past issues.

June was in her early 70s. I hadn't seen her as a patient for four years. I invited her into my office, asking how she had been. Interestingly, she was wearing a tasteful beanie which she kept on throughout the consultation. June informed me that her husband had died three years before and although she was sad, her grieving had stopped long ago. June described the wonderful relationship she'd had with him and that she was content with the memories.

I give a lecture on the speaking circuit, titled, 'Your biography becomes your biology', inspired by the work of Caroline Myss, but also very much based around my own medical practice. I was, however, struggling at the time to find a good example from my own work of a very specific C7 disease.

I asked June why she was wearing the beanie. She removed it to show me a rather large bald spot on the top of her crown, right at the crown chakra. I strongly suspected that June was still living in the past, when her husband was still alive. Her inability to feel content in the present moment was blocking her seventh chakra and, in her case, leading to a substantial loss of hair in this region.

When you have a specific disease, symptoms or purely lack energy, vitality and enthusiasm, it is vital that you view 'mind management' as part of your program. Here are specific tips to maintain the flow in each of your chakras:

C1

The root chakra is also your connection to the earth. Spending time in the garden, bushwalking or swimming in the ocean reconnects you to the earth and it is particularly healing for C1.

C2

Because C2 is the centre of creativity in relationships, it is direct culti-vation of these areas of your life which will keep the energy flow through this centre. Any practice that improves your creativity, such as music, art or writing, is very powerful. Learning a musical instrument, taking that art class or doing a creative writing course are among the suggestions to maintain C2 flows.

Being the area for sex, money and power, it is important, especially if you have C2 symptoms or diseases, that you should focus on your relationships within each of these areas.

Sound financial management is vital. Don't waste your money on goods you don't need. Also, your relationships with the important people in your life are vital to maintain C2 energy flow. Put your effort into the people who will be standing around your bed when you have that heart attack, or those who will be crying at your funeral, because if you don't, they probably won't!

One vital point here is to develop a 'service mentality'. Go into every relationship with the attitude, 'how may I serve?' Make those around you feel special and loved.

C3

With C3 being the centre of personal power, your relationship with yourself is the key here. Although it is a well-worn phrase, it's still very relevant and important – 'If you can't love yourself, you can't love anyone else.' Self care and nurturing are important aspects of energy management.

The great American psychologist Abraham Maslow talks of being a no-limit person. The five aspects of having no limits to your life are as follows:

1. Be independent, with a good opinion of other people. Forget about what other people think of you, it's only what you think that counts. If you base your life on the appraisal or the criticism of others, you're living by their standards, not yours.

2. Be detached from the outcome. Whatever you do, do it because it's right, not for personal or monetary gain.

3. Have no desire for power over others. People who want to dominate other people for any reasons, be it at home, at work or at play, do so because they don't feel enough power within themselves. Anyone who commits domestic violence, bullies or domineering bosses (to give a few examples) have incredibly low self-esteem, and by dominating others they feel that they're gaining this lost power by other means.

4. See beauty in all things. When Mother Teresa was once asked why she helped beggars out of the gutter, she replied, 'It's not between me and the beggar but me and God.' The universal energy of God is everywhere. If you lead a symbolic life you'll be able to see that beauty.

5. Live in the moment. I've mentioned this before, but if you spend your life worrying about mistakes you've made in the past or what may happen in the future, you're detracting from what is happening right now.

C4

Your heart chakra is the centre of your emotions. It is here that the energy of unconditional love has its power. If you ever wish to seek revenge on anyone who has harmed you, turn that around and cultivate forgiveness.

In *Anatomy of the Spirit*, Caroline Myss talks about the concept of woundology. Wearing your past traumas on your sleeve purely keeps the wounds open. Forgiving (regardless of the severity of the harm or trauma) is the most healing act for you, not for the perpetrator of your trauma.

As the law says, love is the ultimate power. Cultivate love, forgiveness and non-judgement.

C5

Being the centre of choice, willpower and decision, this is appropriately located between C4 and C6, i.e. between the heart and the head. Our decisions are therefore a battle between our emotions and our thinking.

Life isn't about making a big decision to be healthy, or to lead a high-quality life; it's about making 30 to 50 small decisions every day. Decisions like, I won't eat that biscuit; I'll walk up the stairs rather than take the escalators; I won't yell at that fool who just cut in front of me in the traffic; I won't have that extra drink of alcohol.

These small decisions either take you towards a good quality, healthy life or the reverse. Think careful about the choices and decisions you make on a moment by moment basis. You can't cultivate this awareness enough.

C6

Being the centre of your thinking, C6 is best managed by you cultivating high-quality thinking. This involves you treating your brain with the utmost respect. Not only does your brain (and your body, for that matter) need high-quality nutrients, it doesn't need low-quality, legal and illegal substances.

Your brain also needs high-quality information through feeding it with exactly that. Try to see every day as an opportunity for learning through reading high-quality books (such as the one you're reading now!); listen to audio CDs or podcasts on a variety of subjects; or enrol in adult education courses or university. Even the daily practice of crosswords or Sudoku or a variety of brain-training courses keep the brain active and your thinking sound.

But this is not just about having your thinking working at its peak, it's also about seeking the truth in all aspects of your life. Live towards your principles in every situation and your sixth chakra will maintain high energy.

C7

This energy centre, the crown chakra, is your direct connection to whatever external source you believe in. If you have religious beliefs, this is your body's portal to God. As I've mentioned, the less religious, but spiritual person might refer to this as universal vibrational energy, whereas atheists might perceive this energy as emanating from nature.

The Indian spiritual teacher Deepak Chopra was once performing a workshop in Australia. In the front row was a man who persistently heckled him throughout the talk. Tiring of the heckling, Deepak asked him, 'Who are you?' The man replied, 'I'm the head of the Australian Sceptics' Association.' Deepak answered, 'I don't believe you!'

So, I'm suggesting C7 is your direct connection to that binding universal, subtle energy that offers you those inspirational 'ah-ha' moments. This energy is the non-measurable glue that supplies the universal intelligence, i.e. making life work in the way it does.

Wayne Dyer once wrote a book titled *You'll See It When You Believe It*. This clever twist of the more typically used phrase illustrates the paradox of life at a spiritual level. When the now-departed billionaire Kerry Packer suffered a cardiac arrest on the polo field and was resuscitated, he stated emphatically, 'There's nothing on the other side!'

He may have been right, but I suspect that for a person who is so enmeshed in the material world it would have taken a considerable time for his 'spirit' to be roused from its enforced slumber – not the few minutes he was in cardiac arrest.

Interestingly, soon after Mr Packer's incident, a beautiful old lady in her 70s came to see me. She said how disappointed she was to find out from Mr Packer that there was no life after death. She went on to tell me that 10 years before, she'd suffered a cardiac arrest, but during the time her heart had stopped, she had the full near-death experience. She experienced the out-of-body looking down on the scene of her resuscitation and then travelled through the tunnel to the light. During this extraordinarily peaceful experience, the light non-verbally communicated to her that it was not her time to die, and she immediately woke up in her body.

I asked her, 'Why don't you consider that your experience was real?'

She replied, 'Because Mr Packer was much more important than I am!' I'll let you all be the judge of that for yourself.

Regardless of culture, religious beliefs, life experiences or personality characteristics, the reality is that around 20 per cent of people who suffer cardiac arrest and are resuscitated have near-death experiences. These people are either lying or the experiences are real.

Modern science tries to explain these in purely scientific terms but can't, probably because science is the exploration of the physical world, not the spiritual world. So, I believe your C7 is the portal to the spiritual world. Again, I realise not everyone will agree, but I believe that this is your direct connection to the divine and to angels (including your guardian angels or spirit guides).

How, then, can you rebalance your energy centres? What techniques can you use in your everyday life that will complete your fifth stage healing process?

Firstly, I suggest you adopt my 'Five D' process for health:

1. Decision

    Firstly, and most importantly, you need to decide what it is that needs to be healed. If you have a specific problem or disease, this decision is quite simple. But you may be lacking energy or feeling a sense of discontent about your life in some other way.

    You need to clearly define what the issues are that you need to resolve and make a strong commitment to yourself to change. A good tip here is to keep a diary or a journal and write down your clear goals. Refer back to this journal, preferably on a daily basis.

Your goal should be: 1. Specific; 2. Measurable; 3. Achievable; 4. Realistic; 5. Time-bounded. As you can see, this is clearly a SMART approach.

2. Direct awareness

This is about developing that observer of your behaviour. As you have now recognised what issues have occurred that have led you to this point in your life, you need to be aware of what aspects of your behaviour continue to promote these issues and what patterns need to be changed.

If, for example, you are someone who needs the approval of others, become aware of how and when you do this, taking conscious steps to avoid these patterns. Remember, see every situation you're in as a test, as a universal decision allowing you to choose what is the best scenario for you to undergo this slow, evolutionary process. Recurring patterns will commonly be presented to you until you have resolved your default reactions.

3. Day to day

As I mentioned earlier, Confucius once said, 'A journey of 1000 steps begins with a single step.' It takes more steps each day to change. For example, if your problem is excessive weight, just cutting down your caloric intake by a small amount every day will have a significant benefit over the course of 12 months.

A loss of only a half a kilogram per week – which is very achievable – amounts to a 26 kilogram weight loss over

12 months, which is very dramatic. Simple habits like walking upstairs, rather than using some mechanical means of movement such as an elevator or an escalator, have a profound long-term effect.

My old office was on the second floor of the building. One of the women working next door to me was morbidly obese. The ground floor was below street level and required walking up 10 steps. But this woman, not wishing to expend any energy, would catch the lift to the first floor where she could take the side door and walk out at street level.

It was no great shock she was morbidly obese!

4. Discipline

In all aspects of life, the most successful people follow one important principle – discipline. I'm not purely referring to financial success, but also success in the physical, mental, emotional and spiritual aspects of your life.

This entire book is about cultivating discipline in all of these areas. Yes, of course, it takes extra effort and, of course, it is easier to cave in and follow the quicker, simple path and, of course, we all fail at different times – but this is the great paradox.

A key point about life is this paradox. What seems quick and easy is usually bad for you and in the long run makes your life harder. What seems a harder and longer path is typically, in the end, better for you and more rewarding.

A number of years ago a study took place in which a group of toddlers were taken into a room and were told they could have a marshmallow straight away, but that if they waited until the person returned, they could have two marshmallows. After this initial experiment, the children were then followed for a number of years until they reached their late teens. There was a clear distinction between those who could exhibit delayed gratification, i.e. wait for the second marshmallow, and those who had to have the marshmallow at the time. Those who could wait for the second marshmallow performed much better at high school, had much greater social skills and were less likely to use drugs of addiction or end up in jail. I must say I believe the researchers who performed this study showed enormous delayed gratification, by waiting close to two decades to obtain the results of their study.

This ability is an enormous aspect of self-discipline. When you have an acute craving for anything – whether this be a substance, a situation, or any type of addicted behaviour – just disciplining yourself to wait for 15 minutes to half-an-hour is a vitally important technique in overcoming this issue. Practise delayed gratification as much as you can in all aspects of your life.

5. Dedication

Any new behaviour or practice that is serving you well has to become an ingrained habit. In his book *Think and Grow Rich*, Napoleon Hill said the greatest success principle is perseverance. I'd actually somewhat change this to say that it is having the discipline to persevere that is the greatest success principle.

Whether it's quitting smoking, losing weight, remembering to take your blood pressure pills or vitamins, or even attending your doctor for follow-up, it requires a lifelong commitment to being healthy.

Earlier, I mentioned the real-estate mantra 'location, location, location'. The good health and healing mantra should be 'persevere, persevere, persevere' with 'discipline, discipline, discipline'. Very simply, rather than seeing your health as a 12-week program that will benefit you for (you guessed it) 12 weeks, see this program as lifelong.

And here are five principles that will help guide your new health plan. I've covered many of these principles throughout the book, but would like to briefly reinforce their importance:

1. Silence

   Spend 30 minutes each day (apart from sleeping) in some form of silence. I'll discuss this further in the section on meditation.

2. Service

   The 'how may I serve' mantra should become a constant in your life. This should include serving yourself through nurturing your physical body, your mind, cultivating healthy emotions, managing your financial affairs and, most importantly, nurturing your soul. You should also serve those most special to you, your acquaintances and the community in general.

3. Law of attraction

   I mentioned earlier in this chapter how your thoughts create your reality. Each thought creates energy and our bodies function on energy. Bad thoughts, and defective thinking and emotions, create defective energy and disrupt the energy flow through our chakras.

Loving, compassionate thoughts, forgiveness and a positive attitude cultivate the same positive energy within our bodies.

4. For the moment

    Yesterday is finished, tomorrow isn't here. This moment is all you ever have. Ensure all your circuits are in present time, thus preventing previous bad habits, life events or collective ancestral beliefs from directing your current energy flows. Be here, now.

5. Balance

    For a variety of reasons, many people in the modern world are out of balance. The Buddhists refer to the 'middle path' of life. This is something we should all strive for. We need to cultivate security but we also need passion. Balance is achieved by following all the advice offered so far in this book in each area: physical, mental, emotional, work life (including financial), and spiritual.

There are five key steps to bring balance into your life:

1. Match your goals with your behaviour

    We all have dreams that we'd like to translate into goals and then into action. I remember as a child enjoying the old style playgrounds which these days would never pass any occupational health and safety standards. I was always the smallest kid in the class and delayed my modest growth spurt until well into my teens. So, in these playgrounds it was difficult for me to find a playmate who could give me a reasonable balance on the see-saw. Thus, I spent most of my time up in the air.

However, this is precisely what matching your goals with your behaviour means. Dreams are said to be the seedlings of reality and the imagination is the fire from heaven. But how many of us go through life cultivating bad habits such as overeating, avoiding exercise and plunging into subtle and not-so-subtle forms of addictions? In the meantime, how many of us lament those behaviours and wish to change? Hence, the symbolic New Year's resolutions. I'd venture to say that people who don't make New Year's resolutions didn't need to in the first place. Reconnect your life behaviour with your dreams, genuine desires and goals.

Addiction is a good example of behaviour conflicting with your dreams and goals. Author Wayne Dyer has introduced a psycho-spiritual approach to resolving addictions. He suggests the following approach:

1. Make the decision for wellbeing
    Realign your desires for this worthy goal. Dr Dyer suggests the silent prayer, 'Make me an instrument of thy wellbeing.'

2. Live the symbolic life
    See your journey through addiction as a great teacher. This has taught you what it is you no longer wish to be. Be grateful for the experience and lessons your addiction has given.

3. Love yourself

   Be grateful for your body and mind. See yourself as being worthy of a new life without your addiction.

4. Remove all shame from your life

   As I've said, life is perfect in its imperfection. You needed this experience in order to move to a higher place.

5. Live from a new knowing

   Your body is pure, now that you live in this addiction-free space.

You also need to rebalance your attitudes to eating and exercise. As you cultivate the observer in your life, have this observer instruct your body to convert all the food you consume into healthy, happy cells. The more you do this, the less you'll feel like consuming unhealthy food. On an equally positive note, develop the same attitude to exercise. Every time you exercise, reinforce the enormous positive good this is doing to your body.

2. Slow down

   How many of us constantly feel we're on this endless treadmill called life? So many people go through the drudgery of the five-day working week to end up with a Friday night wind down (often alcohol fuelled), with a less than restful weekend to start the whole cycle the following Monday.

   One third of the population have stress-related symptoms and/or are taking some form of medication to treat their issues. We are being constantly bombarded by the instant access world. Our mobiles are always switched on and we're constantly checking our emails, either on the ever-present computer or hand-held device. Technology has not made our life any easier; in fact, it's so much harder because of this constant need for the instant response. There is an excellent saying, 'The more you advance towards God, the less he'll give you worldly duties.' In other words, the more you live life through spiritual not material principles, the less need you have to pursue the material aspects of your life.

3. Abundance versus absence

    You become what you think and feel about yourself. If you're primed to think and feel that you're missing something, either by your ancestral DNA or life experiences, and you continue to believe it – you've guessed it, this absence will continue to show up in your life. Think, feel and cultivate abundance. Behave as if you're already there.

4. Choose peace and love

    If you switch on any news service you'll hear, see or read about the evil in the world. This may be suffering through natural disasters, violence or treachery. Wayne Dyer makes the following vital points: 'To see and listen to the wicked is already the beginning of wickedness.' 'All good is from God, all evil is from yourself.' 'Stop watching and involving yourself in this transmitted evil. If we don't give it attention it won't happen.'

5. Experience heaven on earth

    This reinforces my point about living a symbolic life. See heaven in every day of your life. If you lose your emphasis on the material aspects of life, I promise that you'll experience that feeling of balance. The material world is all about stuff. The more stuff you own, the more you win, the more success-ful you are. This is purely another form of addiction, i.e. the more you have, the more you want.

Just when I wanted an example of experiencing heaven on earth, the universe presented it to me in a very simple moment. As I was writing this, it was the hottest February day in Sydney for around 90 years, with the temperature hitting about 42 degrees Celsius. My first grandchild, Edie, was two weeks old, and her mother – my beautiful daughter Bridget – didn't want Edie to suffer the extreme heat, so they stayed the night in our air-conditioned house.

Bridget brought Edie downstairs and she was slightly unsettled. I held this beautiful little angel in my arms and she fell asleep. I valued the opportunity to experience this piece of heaven on earth. Try to see that every moment a living organism is connected energetically. See every accident, tragedy or disaster as part of that connection and ask symbolically what these are trying to teach you. Also, appreciate and value the grace that the universal force is offering.

So, apart from everything I have written up to this point regarding each of these five stages of health, I'd like to finish with the five Ms:

1. Meditation
   One way of healing that I think is incredibly helpful and powerful is meditation. Our specific energetic healing should

be performed by meditating on a daily basis. I've been meditating daily since 1994. To start with, I was taught transcendental meditation, but I've since modified this to incorporate chakra healing. The chakras are arranged from C1 to C7.

I start my meditation session by yoga breathing, which, although it takes a bit of practice, is actually quite simple. I then move on to 20 minutes of mantra meditation based around transcendental meditation. Then I finish off with a five-minute gratitude meditation. This is how I start each day and it is a vital aspect of my life.

Regardless of whether you're trying to heal a specific disease or symptom, or whether you're trying to overcome other significant issues in your life, incorporating meditation into your daily lives is one of the most vital healing techniques. I believe we all need at least half-an-hour off the 'merry-go-round of life' and I certainly suggest that meditation is the best technique to accomplish this.

2. Music

The healing power of music has long been discussed. Professor Luciano Bernadi from the University of Pavia in Italy has performed very elegant studies regarding the ability of musical compositions with a 10-second cycle to align various body rhythms for optimal function.

The brain, the heart and the lungs work on this cycle. When we're sick or stressed, this cycle speeds up as a consequence of the stress. Listening to music with a 10-second cycle can help restore the body rhythms back to this healing cycle.

Professor Bernadi has found that certain compositions from Beethoven, Puccini, Verdi and other classical composers have the ability to heal at this 10-second cycle. Interestingly, some non-classical music compositions have a similar cycle, such as Indian ragas and even one of the compositions from the Red Hot Chili Peppers! The *Ave Maria* in Latin also has a specific 10-second cycle and much of the research was performed around this particular piece.

It may not be too far away when we see these various compositions being suggested as part of a health program.

3. Massage

Whether you're a newborn baby or closer to the other end of life, most of us enjoy and need human touch. I often say a simple principle of life that would stop many of the world's traumas is that if you haven't been invited into someone else's personal space, you have no right to be there. But if you wish to invite someone into your personal space and they comply, this can lead to a number of positive emotions and the release of healthy physiological chemicals.

Taking the sexual aspect out of this discussion (which in itself can lead to all of the above), therapeutic touch, in all its forms, can have multiple healing benefits. There is a variety of forms of massage and I personally have had some type of therapeutic massage, at least fortnightly, for the past 25 years. If you're in a position to use these various therapeutic techniques, these can be an excellent component of your health program.

4. Medicine

You might be surprised that I've included this in the mind health section when I've extensively covered orthodox medicine elsewhere in the book. I'd like to reinforce the importance of integrative medicine; in other words, combining the best aspects of orthodox medicine with the added benefits of aspects of complementary medicine.

However, there is another healing component that I feel isn't emphasised enough – the healing nature of the therapeutic relationship, i.e. your relationship with your doctor or other medical advisor. Having contact and regular follow-up with a trusted health professional is also part of the healing process.

5. Miracles, the mystical and magic

Regardless of your core beliefs, there is something miraculous about the entire process of life. With all its flaws, faults, accidents, tragedies and disasters, there is still a certain order to how the universe functions. Even putting aside the difficulties we have in explaining religious miracles, purely the miracle of birth is astounding.

Throughout the years there have been many people who have been called mystics. They often come from India, but also from elsewhere: native Americans – for instance – also have Shamanistic practices. Many cures and healings have been attributed to mystics from various cultures.

If true mystics with healing power do exist – and it is certainly difficult to explain many of the stories, which have had varying degrees of medical verification – they have been given a bad name by the charlatans and so-called faith-healers seen in some bizarre religions.

Finally, we all know that modern forms of magic are illusion used to entertain. But many of our myths, legends and rituals speak to the core of our basic archetypes and the magic that emanates, symbolically, I believe in some way has healing properties.

Conclusion

The basic aim of every living organism is to survive. But, in our modern world, it's about living longer and living better. To achieve a better quantity and quality of life it is important to understand the basic premises of life and how our modern world often negatively impacts on these foundations.

Our physiology was designed for a natural environment and a shorter lifespan but we now exist in a world affected by synthetic chemicals, man-made sources of radiation and the ever-present chronic stress, all for a much longer time.

The combination of genetic predisposition, the above factors and a whole host of well described other contributing issues have created the modern killers of cardiovascular diseases, cancer and the other illnesses that have emerged over the last century.

Throughout the book I have referred to the macrocosm and the microcosm. If you believe in a grand design or a pure science-based evolution, it doesn't deny the fact that there is a pattern common at both levels. Our bodies function well as a co-operative community with each atom, molecule, cell and organ performing its designated function, interdependently with the components throughout the person.

But equally, these principles work identically with relationships between each other, families, communities and the world at large. Not to mention the solar system, galaxies and the entire cosmos.

This interdependence is an important theme throughout this book. To achieve this ultimate quality and quantity of life we need to avail ourselves of every stage of health.

If you are sick with any significant illness, don't walk away from conventional, orthodox medicine, i.e. Stage 1. But modern medicine focuses on investigating and managing diseases and symptom complexes, and doesn't always look for the why.

Stage 2 examines the factors in your environment that may be contributing to your issues. Are you being exposed to toxic chemicals, both obvious or subtle, which, once discovered and removed from your life, may diminish future risk?

Are there sources of electromagnetic radiation contributing to your current health issues? Don't discount the influence of bad genetics, nor should you feel complacent if both your parents were long livers. Take the test to determine how your genes may have impacted on your health, i.e. make sure you've covered Stage 3.

But, without Stage 4 and 5 interventions, your abnormal health patterns will almost certainly keep recurring. The well-known 17th-century philosopher Rene Descartes made the famous statement, 'I think, therefore I am.' Without a strong consideration of your emotions and your mental processing of such, these factors will continue to impact on your health and your life.

A major concept I am asking you to take from this book (if you haven't already done so) is to create a solid foundation of lifestyle principles – but also have appropriate medical assessments to gauge your current and potential health risks.

The vast majority of this book is based on strong medical science, albeit from, at times, a different perspective. Towards the end of the book, I have presented a somewhat new and, I would suggest, challenging view of how illnesses arise and how to incorporate Stage 5 strategies to, hopefully, facilitate healing.

I present a concept of God as an internal, vibrational energy. I would like to finish with a few explanatory points to clarify my position. Firstly, I have absolutely no proof for this hypothesis – it is purely that. Secondly, I am not being exclusive of any specific religion(s) by those suggestions. It is my opinion that science is only as good as its 'testing' equipment and although our current scientific technology is more sophisticated than at any other time in history, there is still much more to discover and understand, and thus with our present scientific approaches, validation of this proposal is just not possible. Thus it remains purely a hypothesis.

All science begins with hypothesis, some eventually discounted, although many proven. My hypothesis offers an explanation that I believe may be part of the missing link in understanding the potential, deeper reasons as to how illnesses arise, as well as suggested, additional strategies for management.

I have tried to present an integrative approach to health which I believe has to be the way of the future. I would like to finish with my favourite quote that has fuelled my entire life. This was made by the famous painter Michelangelo:

'The greater danger for most of us lies not in setting our aim too high and falling short; but in setting our aim too low, and achieving our mark.'

You can set your aim low and achieve a lesser quality and quantity of life, or you can follow the principles set out in this book, taking your life in a more rewarding, healthier and longer direction.

Bibliography

Books

Dyer, Wayne, *You'll See It When You Believe It*, William Morrow Paperbacks, 2001

Fisher, Donna, *Dirty Electricity*, Joshua Books, 2011

Gray, John, *Men Are from Mars, Women Are from Venus*, HarperCollins, 1992

McLean, Lyn, *The Force*, Scribe Publications, 2011

Myss, Carolyn, *Anatomy of the Spirit*, Three Rivers, 1996

Ruby, Margaret, *The DNA of Healing*, Hampton Roads Publishing, 2006

Smith, Rick, and Bruce Lourie, *Slow Death by Rubber Duck*, UQP, 2009

Journals

BMJ

Cochrane Reviews

The Journal of the American Medical Association

The Lancet

New England Journal of Medicine

New Scientist

Websites

www.abs.gov.au

www.aihw.gov.au

www.cancerscreening.gov.au

www.fightaging.org

www.mayoclinic.com

www.medicalnewstoday.com

www.medlineplus.gov

www.prostate.org.au